DEMENT

John Radzienda

DEMENTIA: A Son's Story
Copyright © 2018 by John Radzienda

All rights reserved. This book or any portion thereof may not be reproduced or used in any manner whatsoever without the express written permission of the publisher except for the use of brief quotations.

These writings are in no way meant to be taken as medical or professional advice and are strictly the author's personal observations passed on to you in this memoir. This book is not intended as a substitute for the medical advice of physicians. The reader should regularly consult a physician in matters relating to his/her health and particularly with respect to any symptoms that may require diagnosis or medical attention.

Produced in the United States of America
ISBN: 978-1-7329528-0-5

Published by:
JFR Publishing

The author can be reached at:
johnradzienda@gmail.com

EARLY SIGNS

My mom, Nancy Radzienda (nee Shanahan), didn't sit still for long and, to put it mildly, she loved to drive. Wherever she went when she was driving, she made a beeline. She knew exactly where she was going and what she wanted to do when she got there and, usually, she didn't drive slowly.

As a teenager in Chicago, when she was learning to drive, her dad frequently told her to "Gun it, Nance!" And that's what she did.

In the summer of 2011, Ma decided she was ready for a new car. She had a mid-sized SUV and she thought she'd like another one. I did a little research and came up with a model with a four-cylinder engine, which seemed a little light, but I felt like it was the safest choice. She would have preferred the six-cylinder, because this would have made it much easier for her when she needed to "gun it."

Right after the purchase, it was time to hit the road. She wanted to take it to Chicago and visit my older brother, Jim, and my younger sister Mary Ann and both of their families. She'd also visit with her sister and brother-in-law, my Aunt Mary and

Uncle Jim. This trip was fine with my brothers and me because, although she had been showing some minor signs of mental decline, there had been no indication that her decision-making abilities had been affected in a harmful way. The next day, well before first light, she was on her way. A bag of donuts, numerous strawberry licorice twists, a couple pounds of cookies, and a cooler loaded with diet soda. Yes, the food provisions were in place.

After many years of these road trips, we always asked her to give us a call on the first night, so we'd know that she'd made it safely. On this particular trip, she called and said, "Oh honey, I've had an accident."

"What! Are you okay? Where are you at?"

"Oh, I'm fine. I'm in eastern Nebraska"

"Well, what happened?"

"I don't know. I was just driving down the Interstate and all of a sudden it felt like I hit something, but I never saw anything and all of a sudden I couldn't control the car very well and I got over on the shoulder and the car just stopped."

"Ma, what do you mean you didn't see anything? It must have been something pretty major to cause the car to come to a halt after doing seventy miles an hour."

"Well I don't know, but there were other people stopped on the shoulder ahead of me, so they must have hit the same thing."

Now, this just didn't sound right to me, but she didn't budge on her story. Of course, my only concern was that she was safe, and it seemed like she was, so I didn't press any further for the details. However, I did notice that I heard kids in the background on her end of the phone. "Ma, I swear I hear kids in the background. Where are you?"

"Oh, I'm at the tow truck driver's house."

My heart skipped a beat and I couldn't talk right away. As soon as my breathing returned to normal, I asked, "How did you get there?"

"Well, he towed my car to the dealer and I didn't see any motels around. He told me that I could stay at his house if I wanted to and I said okay."

"That's it? Are you telling me that a town big enough to have a GMC dealer isn't big enough to have a hotel or motel or bed and breakfast or something?"

Then she took the independent, hardline response, "Well, he's a nice guy and his wife and kids are nice, too."

"But Ma, lots of serial killers are nice guys. How can you possibly think that this is okay?"

She finally had to lay down the law with, "Well it's just fine and that's the end of it. I'll call you tomorrow."

And then she hung up on me. End o' story. After I was able to start talking again, I called my brother Jim in Illinois and asked him if he'd talked to Ma lately. He said, "Yeah, I just talked to her a half hour ago. Sounds like she's roughly equidistant from both of us."

I said, "Well whaddaya think?"

He said, "I think that if either of us left right now, and she is staying with a serial killer, she'd be dead before we got there."

Yep. He was right. If she was just another notch on the gearshift lever in the case of the "Tow Truck Murders," she surely was a goner. I had trouble sleeping that night as I worked through several potential scenarios. Should I have gone to Nebraska? Should I have called the local police department? I always figured I'd get gray hair because of my teenage daughters, not my mother.

The next afternoon, Ma called and said that she'd made it to her sister's house JUST FINE. It all worked out. "I don't know what you were so worried about," she said.

A GOOD SENSE OF DIRECTION

My mom frequently said that she had a good sense of direction and I knew that she could drive anywhere in North America, regardless of which direction she needed to go, and not get lost. I knew this because she did it numerous times over the years. But whenever she was in her basement, for reasons that still baffle me, she had absolutely no idea which wall corresponded to the front of her house. Or which wall corresponded to the back of her house. Given that, I guess she might have had a good sense of direction, but with certain restrictions like, she didn't know which way she was facing when she was in her basement. On one occasion, we were downstairs in the laundry room and I said, "Oh yeah, I forgot to tell you that I put a new downspout on the front of the house, on the southeast corner."

She looked over at the window that was below ground level on the front wall of the house, where she couldn't see anything but a window well. Then she quickly pivoted on one leg and looked in turn at the washer, dryer, laundry tub, hot water heater, and furnace. Then the desk. Then the doorway. Then, near the end of the circle, she saw her sewing cabinet with the fabric falling off the top. Finally, she completed the circle. She was ready to take another lap, but I decided to stop her. She was once again facing the front of the house and said, "I get so twisted around down here."

I'd tease her about it all the time. She had a great sense of humor and we joked with each other back and forth regularly.

She was sharp as a tack (except when it came to basement navigation). At least she had always been sharp as a tack, but as time went on she continued to show more signs of mental decline. For example, my younger brother, Tom, has lived in Thailand for over twenty years. He comes to the States regularly, say, every one to three years. He'll generally be in the country for a couple months, splitting his time between the Chicago area and Colorado Springs. On one of these trips, he was due to arrive in Colorado Springs mid-afternoon. Ma was going to pick him up and bring him over to our house for supper. Around four in the afternoon he called me from the passenger seat in Mom's car. Even though I could tell he was concerned, he casually said, so as not to alarm Ma while she was driving, "I don't live here, but it doesn't seem like we should be heading south on Powers Boulevard after leaving the airport."

I told him that "Of the four main compass directions you could have taken when leaving the airport, East and South would have been equally bad because you would never, ever, have been able to make it to our house. Where are you now?"

He explained where they were, and I gave him directions back to our house from there. When they arrived, I was worried about Ma and asked her what was up. Why did she go south from the airport? She said, "I was looking for the tollway."

I said, "Ma, there isn't a tollway in Colorado Springs."

She did not receive this well and slapped the counter with her hand and in a firm voice said, "Yes there is, I've been on it lots of times."

"Ma, you must be thinking of the Denver airport (DIA is approximately ninety miles northeast of our house). There's a tollway from DIA that takes you south towards Colorado Springs, remember?"

She then slowly backed away from the counter and tried to talk, but nothing came out. Her hand slowly slid off the countertop. She turned away and quit looking at me. She became withdrawn and her general countenance sank as she realized that she'd mixed up the two cities. This was very upsetting for me as well because she had been to the Colorado Spring airport numerous times over the years and knew exactly where it was. The navigational issues that confused her in her basement were now becoming a concern outside of the house as well.

TIME FOR A LITTLE PAPERWORK

Around the time of the airport mishap, Ma started to have issues with handling her finances. This was extremely out of character because she had always been good with numbers and calculations. She entered the workforce when Tom became a first grader in 1969, as she and my dad continued to raise four young kids. We lived in Oak Lawn, Illinois, mainly a blue-collar suburb, southwest of Chicago. She held various office jobs and during this time she also picked up an associate degree in accounting from the local community college. Eventually, she ended up with a position as an office manager at a tool and die manufacturing plant south of Chicago, where she easily managed all the financial recordkeeping and other organizational tasks that this position required. During this period she also became a certified credit union executive.

Because of her education, her career, and her general nature she had always been quite neat, tidy, and accurate with her finances and general record keeping. She balanced the books to the penny because that's the way it's done, thank you very much. She kept her file folders arranged alphabetically by category and, as far as I knew, she was still up to the task. Out of the blue one day, she mentioned that she wanted me to look over "a little paperwork" concerning her bank accounts, CDs, and stocks. Financial stuff. I said, "Sure Ma, just bring it over and we'll take a look."

I thought she'd bring over something like a grocery store plastic bag filled with a few hard-to-understand documents that we'd square away in no time. The next week she came over with three good-sized boxes, each one about as big as four shoeboxes. Huh? Each box was crammed full of all manner of letters, account statements, envelopes, quarterly reports, and junk mail in a real hodgepodge of a mess. A disaster. Three months later, I finally had it all straightened out.

I took over most of her financial affairs from that point on, although she still wanted to take care of her day-to-day banking, which was minimal. Of course that was fine with me, but eventually I'd take that over as well. It was shocking when she eventually admitted, "I just can't do it anymore."

MY MOM, THE TRAVELER

She was upset not only because her financials were overwhelming, but also because she was beginning to realize that she might have issues with the logistics involved with her frequent traveling adventures. She had gone all over the world for decades and it was her favorite leisure activity. I mean she REALLY loved to travel and when Tom moved to Thailand in 1992, she couldn't wait to go to Southeast Asia. Over the next seventeen years she visited Thailand several times and when she was there they'd usually take a trip to Malaysia, or some other location in that part of the world. She rode on an elephant on one of the trips and on another she joined Tom with some of his monk friends for a visit and afternoon tea. They explored all manner of places, from Buddhist temples to small fishing villages on the coast. Sometimes she wouldn't go to Thailand and instead she'd meet Tom, say, in Sri Lanka. There was a trip to Borneo on another occasion.

She had also traveled extensively in Europe as well as in Australia, New Zealand, and Africa, in addition to covering thousands of miles in the States, Mexico, and Canada. She even had the bug as a thirteen-year-old when she and her sister traveled by train from Chicago to Montana to visit with relatives on a cattle ranch just east of Livingston.

She and my dad dated the last two years of high school and a few years after that, in January 1957, they were married. Less than one year later, Dad was drafted and entered the U.S. Army. After his training period he went to his permanent station in Nurnberg, Germany where he and Ma lived for just over a year. This was just long enough for my older brother, Jim, to be born outside of the U.S.

Before she relocated from Illinois to Colorado, she had previously made many trips to visit my wife Sandy and me. We went backpacking, hiking, fishing, and white-water rafting. She was a real trouper and never let anything as trivial as a 6,000 to 9,000-foot elevation gain get in her way of enjoying the Rocky Mountains.

Sometimes she traveled alone, sometimes with a relative or friend, and other times it'd be an organized tour. She'd been from New Zealand to Russia to Hawaii to Bangladesh, and many other places in between. Don't forget Peru and Argentina when Tom lived there for a year.

Starting in 2000, five years after my dad passed away, she retired from her job in Illinois and began her career as a part-time volunteer for the National Park Service, at the Golden Gate Recreation Area in northern California. She returned there every January for three months, over the course of twelve years. When volunteering in California, she worked in the office area and bunked in a room in a large house out in the woods.

And she was enamored with Alaska. She'd driven there by herself, more than once, and slept in her car when necessary. She went with her sister and brother-in-law on one occasion and she was always looking for another reason to go there again. She loved the old mining towns and the opportunity to take a ton of photos of the beautiful scenery and wildlife. Whether by land, sea, or air, she was always up for a trip to our northernmost state, or just about anywhere else.

The girl got around.

Because of all this traveling, she'd been in many airports around the world. She was a seasoned travel vet who knew just where she kept her itinerary, ticket, and boarding passes. Lip balm was here, cell phone was there, and she kept her ever-present candy stash in more than one location and she knew right where it all was. She'd be dressed nicely, usually in her trademark turquoise and green outfit of some sort, always with matching earrings, and she was quite adept at dealing with any obstacle that came her way. In advance, she knew where she was staying on each night of her journey.

Then one day, at the start of one of her trips, she asked my wife Sandy to give her a ride to the airport. Usually, we'd drop her off at the terminal door and she'd quickly exit the car, have a quick hug, grab her bag and shoot inside the airport like a rocket, "See ya when I get back!" she'd shout over her shoulder. Small talk and long goodbyes were not necessary. On this trip though, she asked Sandy if she could come inside the airport with her. When they walked through the main doors of the airport, Ma stopped, looked around, turned to Sandy and asked, "What do I do?"

And she meant it. This was quite shocking because she truly didn't know what to do. This is from a woman who had spent countless hours in airports all around the world. Sandy went through the motions with her and she managed to get on the plane and jet off to wherever she was going. The rest of her trip went off without a hitch, but this was a very noticeable sign that all was not well with our world traveler.

I began to notice more and more changes in her behavior. They were little things that an adult would notice about their mom, even if they weren't apparent to anyone else. I called the doctor's office a few times and explained these things that my mom was doing that were out of character for her. The nurse took notes and said, "Let's see if we can get her in for some testing." And they did just that, more than once.

She'd take a test with a psychiatrist of some sort and the results would come back AOK. In addition, the doctors were able to observe my mom's behavior during her office visit and you can believe that she did whatever she could to prove that she was fine. She was determined to prove that she could continue to live life on her own terms and I sure couldn't fault her for that. I don't know exactly what she did, but, at a minimum, I expect that she aggressively denied the notion of any unusual behavior on her part. I assumed this was the case because that's what she did when she was with me! So that, and whatever else she did during these tests, worked, because the results said that she was JUST FINE.

Sure.

ROYAL FLUSH

We began to keep a closer eye on her. We tried to determine which of her behaviors were due to "old age," and which of them were not. It was frequently difficult to distinguish between the two but there's no doubt that, mentally, she was slipping. The initial indications of her decline were mainly events that occurred in locations other than her house. The basement navigation phenomenon was in the house of course, but that was just one of her funny peculiarities that had gone on for years. Then, one night after work, I received a panicked phone call, "Honey, please come over and plunge my toilet. It's clogged and the water's up to the top."

I explained, "Ma, it's nine o'clock at night, I've had a couple glasses of wine and I just got out of the shower after being gone for thirteen hours at work and I'm whooped. Does the downstairs toilet work?"

"Yeah, as far as I know."

"Is everything okay other than the plugged upstairs toilet?"

"I guess so," she said.

"Then Sandy or I will be over tomorrow to plunge 'er out. Gravity may win, and the clog may free itself. Until then, just use the basement toilet, okay?"

And then she hung up on me.

I couldn't believe it! It wasn't the first time in recent memory where she would lose her temper very quickly when things weren't how she expected them to be. Now, we all have the capacity to lose our temper and we all know that we like things a certain way, that's understood, but it was now different with her. She was usually easy-going for as long as I could remember, but suddenly she had become increasingly quick to get upset over seemingly trivial matters.

The next day she called and informed me that I didn't need to worry about the toilet anymore. I asked her how it cleared up and she said that she saw some guy walking down the street and asked him if he could come in and plunge her toilet. You heard me right. She asked a complete stranger to come into her house and do this. In the guy's defense, he must have been extremely nice. She told me this, and it's hard to know for sure, but I think she was exerting her independence and rubbing it in my face just a bit.

I had previously lived in the same area several years before, so I knew the neighborhood well and felt it was a great place for her. It was comprised of older houses on wide, tree-lined streets. There were your standard ranch style houses along with tri-levels and bi-levels; her house was a red brick rancher with white trim and a carport in front of the one car garage. The location was generally peaceful and safe, and the people were friendly. Apparently, they were even nicer than I remembered. This wasn't the first time she'd had clogged toilet issues for no apparent reason, so I asked her, "Ma, are you putting anything unusual down the toilet?"

"Just pee and poop," she said.

A couple days later, I was at her house and checked the flush on the toilet and it went off without any problems. So, what was she putting down the toilet? At least that's what I was thinking. Within a couple weeks it clogged again, and this time I called a professional. They ran an auger down the line and came up with nothing. The pipes were clean. I was at work at the time and called over to her house while this was going on, told the guy the whole story, then asked him if he could go the extra mile and really check out the drain and P-trap plumbing that's internal to the toilet and all that. He called me back thirty minutes later, "Got 'er!"

I was on the edge of my seat, "What'd you find?"

"A rag."

"Huh?"

"A rag. A washrag. There was a rag stuck in the P-trap in her toilet! Apparently, sometimes it would block the drain and other times it wouldn't. It could definitely cause an intermittent flushing problem."

I couldn't help myself and teased Ma, "I guess when I asked you what you were putting down the toilet and you said, 'Just pee and poop,' you should've said, 'just pee and poop and a rag.'"

Right after I said that, I had a flashback to when my youngest daughter was three years old. One day she came out of the bathroom with a big smile on her face and proudly announced that she had just flushed her shirt down the toilet. I told her that that was not a good thing to do and that nothing goes down the toilet but pee and poop. We didn't have any issues with the drains backing up, so I assumed the t-shirt had made it out to the main sewer line.

A couple weeks later, I went down into my crawlspace and discovered hundreds of gallons of "dirty" wastewater. Oh no! I brought my daughter down there and showed her why we don't flush shirts down the toilet and she said, "Okay Daddy."

Her work was finished and mine had just begun. I removed a few floating boxes that had been in the wrong place at the wrong time and then called in the pros. After the cleanup, it was time for the drain guy to run his snake down the nasty sewer line and retrieve the shirt. He had to go on the roof and access the drain from a vent pipe because that was the only way it would work. Sandy and I were down on the ground watching and eventually he said, "I think I got it!"

And with that, he held up this indistinguishable gob. My wife yelled up to him, "Is it orange and yellow?"

He said, "Kinda," and tossed it down for us to inspect.

Things then returned to normal and stayed that way for about a week until I discovered that my daughter had somehow managed to flush a pencil down another toilet. After that, there weren't any further issues with the perpetual potty-plugger, and I never gave it any further thought until the incident with my mom. I didn't recall having any issues with toilet non-flushables myself, even when I was a kid, so if this is a genetic trait, it had apparently skipped a generation.

THE GREAT ESCAPE

While we're on the subject of toilets, it's worth mentioning that Ma was beginning to intermittently have a hard time standing up after using the toilet. Couches and chairs weren't an issue, but the toilet sometimes gave her grief, probably because it was so low. Eventually, she started having more and more problems with her back, hip, and right leg. The pain was getting worse and it was really bothering her in January 2012. She never complained about her health very much, so when she brought this up frequently, I knew it needed attention. I don't recall if it was sciatica or not, but it was surely a nerve issue, caused by a narrowing of the spinal cord opening where the nerves passed through and this caused undue pressure on the nerves and, hence, the pain. Because of this, she had surgery to enlarge the opening through which the nerves passed.

In her past, she gave birth to four kids. My brother Jim, born in Germany, is the oldest. He lives south of Chicago with his wife and two kids in their

twenties. I'm next in line and live in Colorado Springs with my wife and two teenage kids. Mary Ann is our sister and she's next in line age-wise. She also lives south of Chicago with her husband and one of their kids who's in his twenties. They have three other kids, two who live in Austin, Texas and the other near Milwaukee. Tom, my youngest sibling, has lived abroad for over twenty-five years and currently lives near Chiang Mai, Thailand with his wife.

She had also been in the hospital after a bad car accident in 1971 but, other than that, she hadn't really spent much time in a hospital and certainly hadn't undergone any major surgeries.

She was gung-ho about the operation, but I don't think she fully understood what was coming. I believe she expected to have the operation, recoup for a couple days, and then get back to business as usual.

The operation was a success - no surprises and the doctor was pleased. Unfortunately, the surprises came AFTER the surgery. Initially, they figured that she'd be in the hospital for ten days or so but, in reality, it turned out to be closer to three weeks. The physical therapists wanted her to walk, but she wouldn't. Exercises? No way. It hurt, and she just didn't know how to deal with it. She was not a good patient.

At one point, the head nurse explained that they might have to move her to a nursing home because they could only keep her in the hospital for so long. If she didn't cooperate, they'd have no choice. I had a long talk with her and explained how it was going to hurt for a while and that she needed to do what they said. Anything to get her moving. Did I mention that she wasn't a good patient?

One Saturday morning during this episode, my family and I were having a late breakfast when Sandy received a text from one of my nieces, "Did you know that Gramma tried to escape from the hospital last night? She said that she had left Uncle John (me) a couple voice messages on his cell phone."

Now, as a rule, I turn my cell phone off before I go to bed, so it was off on this particular morning. I retrieved my phone, quickly turned it on and this is the message I had waiting for me from two a.m.: "Hi honey, don't call me back. There's something radically wrong with this….place. I gotta get outta here. Don't call me back. Just come with your car and we'll get everything that we can. Bye bye."

There was another message at four thirty a.m.: "Hi honey. Please come and get me. I don't know where to tell you I'm at. Please come and get me. Bye bye."

After listening to these messages, I hurried over to the hospital to see how Houdini was making out. As I sat in the lobby waiting for her to finish her physical therapy, she went walking by with the physical therapist. It was more of a shuffle than a walk, but she was recovering from major back surgery so that wasn't unusual. As I watched her without her noticing that I was there, I just couldn't believe that the woman walking down the hallway was my own mother. She looked to be in a daze and was only moderately aware of her surroundings as she slowly moved down the hall. She was actually walking which, in this context, was certainly a step in the right direction (pun intended). It was shocking to see my independent mom in her hospital gown and barely able to make it down the hallway, even with someone helping her. It's certainly not that she was doing anything wrong, it's just that this was so uncharacteristic of her. When she went around the corner and out of sight, I started talking to the nurses at their station and they filled in a bunch of the missing pieces for me. It turned out that not only had Ma called me in the middle of the night, but she had also called 911. Twice.

The nurses, and then a doctor, proceeded to tell me about the condition called sundowning, sundowners, or sundowner's syndrome. It's a symptom of dementia and those who experience this tend to become confused, agitated, and restless. Memory loss can also increase during these episodes. The term "sundowners" refers to the fact that these behaviors tend to surface in the evening, while the sun is setting, and continue throughout the night. The doctor went on to explain that certain medications, especially pain medications, could cause a sundowning response. In addition, it was common for it to happen when a person was in an unfamiliar location, such as a hospital. They were all quite sure that this is what happened to Ma, and it seemed logical to me as well. I didn't know it at the time, but this was more or less the point at which my education began.

When she made it back to her room, we talked for quite a while and she still seemed confused and was quite adamant that, "There's something wrong with this place."

As the days went on and her physical therapy continued, she finally began to show signs of returning to her pre-operation self. But she didn't come all the way back. This happened more than once during the coming months: No matter what trauma she went through, be it physical or mental, she never quite fully recovered to the pre-trauma state. Instead, it was evident that she was gradually going down a staircase of declining physical and mental health. In retrospect, the hospital stay was the unofficial beginning of her descent into dementia.

On one of her last nights in the hospital, a social worker came by to check on her mental condition. She asked Ma, "Nancy, have you felt depressed recently?"

Ma firmly stated, "No. No, I've never had any of that although there has been a little bit of it in my family." She then looked at me, for confirmation.

Hmmm. Not true. Ma had shown several signs of depression in the past but never seemed willing to confront it, except in casual tones and then she'd dismiss it quickly. I, along with my wife and siblings, had known for years that she suffered from bouts of depression and anxiety.

Eventually, Ma finished painting a picture of her solid mental health to the social worker, Karen. In her mind, she had proven that she was mentally sound. I then asked Karen if we could talk in private. "Of course," she said.

I spoke with her for thirty minutes and explained all the various issues we'd seen with Ma. I explained how, for the last few months, we could never get any kind of official diagnosis indicating that she was declining in a manner that was something more than "old age." The social worker understood all this and explained that she was not really in a position to do much more than make suggestions as to how we should proceed.

That is, until I brought up the issue of driving. As I mentioned previously, Ma had not given me a reason to take her keys just yet, although the mysterious accident during the "Tow Truck Driver Scandal" had certainly raised my awareness level. Karen informed me that there was a driving test that Ma could take and that this would determine her overall driving condition. Yes! I asked Karen to have the doctor prepare the necessary paperwork that would require Ma to undergo the driving evaluation before she could drive long distances again.

On the day before her discharge from the hospital, I was in Ma's room and we were getting her things packed. She was antsy, and it was nice to see her getting back into her all-business mode. There was one bag filled and ready to go and it was on the bed while we talked to the nurse on duty. As soon as the nurse left the room, Ma handed me several boxes of tissues, along with a few cartons of Ensure and whispered in an urgent tone, "Here. Put these in the bag, underneath my clothes."

I explained that she had already paid for these items and it wasn't necessary to conceal them. But she insisted, and when the nurse came back in the room Ma played it beautifully and, although she didn't say it, she acted as if there was "nothing out of the ordinary going on here."

While all this hospital business was going on, Sandy came up with the idea that maybe she should quit her job, or at least cut her hours back, then Ma could move in with us and we'd just take care of her full time as she grew older. After her release from the hospital, when she came to stay with us for a couple weeks, we decided to use that as a trial run to see if this was a valid notion. It didn't take long to realize that this had been a bad idea. It was hard to believe that there was no way that we could have my mom staying with us full time, but her lifestyle was very incompatible with ours and the thought of Sandy acting as a caregiver dissipated as quickly as it came.

During this two-week period, my mom had the first part of her driving evaluation. I took her to the testing area over at the hospital, and after I made sure she was in good hands I left for a couple hours until the end of the class. When I arrived to pick her up, I walked through the front door and could see her standing in the lobby in her baby blue sweat suit. She was pacing. And she was pissed.

I thought it best to talk to the instructor because she could fill me in with the details. In short, Ma had failed several portions of the test. They said that based on these results it would be fine if she drove on her own as long as she stayed in town, but no more long-distance trips. She also needed to take another portion of the test in a couple weeks. She would actually drive during this test and afterwards they'd be able to give us their final analysis of my mom's driving situation.

Several days after this first test, I brought her and her suitcase to her house. She was then back on her own again and able to drive for the time being. I must admit that I was glad that it looked like she wouldn't be able to drive much in the future, although we still had to wait for the second part of the test. To be clear, she had not really done anything that I was aware of that would indicate she was a danger on the road. I just wanted to do my best to stop her from driving before it got to that point. I could have simply taken her keys, but I didn't feel that it was time for that just yet.

> **This reminded me of 1975, when I was 16. My mom's dad had been steadily declining mentally, and one day grandma made the call to my mom and said, "It's time to take the car from papa."**
>
> **My mom took me with her so that I could drive her car back home. She was visibly upset and not happy at all about having to take the keys from my grampa and drive his car away. "I don't like this," she said, "I don't like this one bit!" She never yelled much, but she yelled then. She calmed down and continued, "One day you guys will be taking the keys from me, and you won't like it either."**
>
> **At the time, I didn't grasp why it was such a hard thing for my mom, but I sure understood it when history repeated itself. I didn't like it either. As a side note, grampa's car that we brought home that day eventually became my first car, a couple years later. A 1972 Dodge Dart with a V-8. I gunned it too.**

The driving-test day arrived, and they said Ma could use her own car for the test, which seemed like a good idea to me. When it was over, I met with the instructor and she gave me the lowdown. She said that Ma did surprisingly well, although she could have paid more attention to the road. It turned out that Ma felt it was her duty to act as a tour guide and she pointed out several local attractions during the test, as opposed to paying strict attention to the road. Other than that, she did pretty well. In short, the evaluator said that their final suggestion was that Ma should only drive around town and only during daylight hours. No more highway driving and no more long trips. Then I found out that this testing agency had no connection to the Department of Motor Vehicles in any way, shape, or form; they had no official power to mandate that she do anything. All they could do was make suggestions and provide the test results to my mom's primary care doctor. Then it would be up to the doctor to decide the outcome.

It had a dubious odor.

The next week I went to her doctor appointment with her and Ma started the appointment with, "If I can't drive, it'll kill me."

The doctor read the driving test report in a casual manner, disregarded it in an equally casual manner and said, "You drive just fine."

I couldn't believe my ears because the doctor had never been in a car with my mom in his life. I couldn't believe that we had spent hundreds of dollars on an evaluation that carried no weight whatsoever. In addition, if she had been so inclined, she could have jumped in her car RIGHT THEN and drove through the night towards Alaska. What the?

THE EYE OF A PHOTOGRAPHER

Because of the driving test not resulting in any definitive changes to Ma's driving habits, she was able to continue driving for the time being and she still talked of traveling on a regular basis. So, I'll move on to another interest of hers that she loved and participated in regularly. Photography. Oh yeah. She loved the finesse and artistic nature of photography for decades. This, along with her love of sewing and playing the piano (not at the same time), allowed her to use her more artistic side where she could be more creative and give her methodical, logical side a break. More than one person had told her that she "had an eye for it," and she did. Her father had been a photographer and his entire working career had revolved around photography.

Here's a short clip from the flyer at his retirement party:

> **Shanahan was a former freelance photographer who competed with the best of Chicago's newspaper photographers during the Roaring 20's and 30's at the scenes of fires, explosions, and other hectic events.**

Apparently, she had inherited his love of, and talent for, photography. My siblings and I have several of her photographs on display in our homes. In my bedroom alone, I have three beautiful examples. One is a shot taken in an African village. It's a close-up of a herd of goats moving down a dusty road between two huts. She used color film, but the setting is such that it's mainly in various shades of black and white, except for the two tribesmen near the center of the photo in their bright red shirts. Photo number two focuses on an elderly woman working on the grounds of an ancient palace in Thailand. It shows two fires used for burning the yard waste and most of the photo shows the plumes of white smoke and the woman raking around the fires. She's in front of one of the plumes and it looks like she magically appeared out of the smoke, like a genie. Number three is a black and white shot of Monument Valley on the Arizona/Utah border – it looks like a promotional photo from a John Wayne movie.

She certainly took some wonderful photos, that's a fact. Her boyfriend Bill was, and still is, an avid photographer and, as a result, they took several trips that revolved around photography in one way or another.

Bill and Ma initially met on one of her many trips, and after that they stayed in touch. He's several years older than her and is a retired engineer from Los Angeles. The intelligence that had served him so well during his working career is still very evident, and he has many varied interests in addition to photography. He's been out to Colorado many times, even though the altitude gives him, and his pacemaker, grief. He's a wonderful, kind, and generous man that always treated my mom, and my family, very well. Of all the people I know, he's the closest I have to a father figure in my life. He's also the closest person my kids have to a grandfather figure in their lives.

Early in the fall of 2012, Bill heard about a photographic seminar in Estes Park, CO, which is one of the gateways to Rocky Mountain National Park and is approximately 140 miles north of Colorado Springs. He couldn't make it, but he thought it'd be worth my mom's time if she went up and checked it out. Ma then called and asked me to go over the map with her, which we did a couple days later. She just needed to take I-25 north from Colorado Springs until she came to Highway 34 near Loveland (120 miles). Taking this left turn would then take her right into Estes Park. It may not have been the shortest or quickest route, but it was surely a very easy, direct path to take. Now, she was fine with all that, but she still wanted me to go over the map with her. She hesitated in her speech when we talked about the route and she seemed quite disinterested in the whole thing. This was very much out of character for her, given her love of traveling and photography. I showed her the route on the map and traced it with a highlighter so that she could easily see that it was a one-turn trip. But she fidgeted constantly and stepped away from the table several times as we discussed the route. It became increasingly clear to me that she did not want to make the trip. Not at all.

My traveler was terrified.

She had driven all over Europe with Tom several times and spent nearly fifty years of her driving life negotiating the streets in and around Chicago. She had gunned her way all over North America and places beyond, but now she was very concerned about this relatively short trip to Estes Park. What was happening to my mom?

I explained to her that I'd need to talk to the people that were hosting the event and that they could provide the best directions as to how to proceed to their location once she arrived in Estes Park. It seemed like a done deal. Completely out of the blue, ten days before the trip, she called me and said, "Oh honey, I've fallen and hit my head on the doorknob."

"What! Holy cow Ma, are you okay?"

"I'm fine. But I think I need to cancel that trip to Estes."

"Do you need to go to the hospital? Are you bleeding or throwing up? Why do you need to cancel the trip?"

"I just don't feel good about going up there."

I went right over to her house to check on her and she had a puffy, red area forming around the eye where she'd hit the doorknob on the way down. She explained to me the events that occurred during the fall and, although somewhat unusual, it certainly could've happened how she described.

The next day I stopped and saw her after work and by then the black eye had arrived. She then handed me a camera and said, "Here, take a picture of my face."

"What's that for, Ma?"

"So I can send it to Bill and he can see that I'm not making anything up."

"Sounds good, Ma."

SUNDOWNER'S AT SEA

In the late fall of 2012, after recovering from her run-in with the doorknob, Ma was going on a cruise to Hawaii with Bill and another couple. She wanted to drive to Bill's house, north of Los Angeles, rather than fly. Why she preferred to drive all the way to L.A., but was afraid to drive to Estes Park, mystifies me to this day. Maybe she was concerned about the photography seminar being too hard to handle?

At any rate, after she arrived at Bill's house, they had a couple days to visit before they were to board the cruise ship and head to Hawaii. Ma called me from Bill's to let me know that she'd made it to California in good shape. She had a lot of fun on the cruise, the weather was wonderful, and she enjoyed the people that she met. On the day that she was supposed to be back in L.A., I received a call from my brother Jim, "Have you talked to Ma today?" he asked.

"No, not yet. I figured I'd call her tomorrow after she'd had a good night's sleep."

"Well, I just called Bill's to check on her and she's there, but she's really sick and had some kind of medical problems on the boat."

I got off the phone with Jim and called Bill right away and he explained that Ma got sick on the last day of the cruise. Bad cough, sore throat, and a fever. He took her to the ship's doctor who then prescribed cough syrup with codeine or some such. After her previous experience with medication, and the sundowner's episode at the hospital, I was afraid of what Bill was going to tell me next.

"We went to bed and, in the middle of the night, I got up to use the restroom. When I came back to the bed it dawned on me that Nancy was gone! I was temporarily shocked, but then there was a knock at the cabin door. It was the friend of mine that we were traveling with, and Nancy, in her nightgown!"

As it turned out, Ma had gotten up to use the bathroom but went through the wrong door and ended up in the ship's hallway. Bill's friend had been up for some late-night gambling and just happened to run into Ma as she was wandering the halls. Bill told me that she had made an honest mistake because the bathroom door and the main cabin door were right next to each other. Apparently, she meant to enter the bathroom and ended up in the hallway instead. There were no further issues on the boat and they made it back to Bill's house with no problems.

After Bill told me the above story, Ma was awake and able to talk on the phone. She sounded just awful because she was very sick and weak, but she was able to talk for a few minutes and assure me that she was fine. A couple days after that she still didn't feel well enough to drive, so Bill drove her, in her car, to Colorado and then he caught the train a week later to go back to L.A.

While Bill was in Colorado, he had trouble breathing due to the altitude. He had the pacemaker I mentioned above, but he'd also lived at sea level all his life, so he was used to plenty of oxygen in the air. For whatever reason, as Ma got better during his stay, she decided it was time to take a trip up to the mountains, higher than the approximately 6000-foot altitude of Colorado Springs where Bill was already having breathing problems. I suggested that maybe she ought to stay around town, but she had it set in her mind that they were heading for the hills. They had a nice day trip but, later that night, she had to take Bill to the hospital emergency room due to breathing difficulties. I said, "It probably would have been better if you had stayed at home instead of going to the mountains."

She said, "It's all right, he has an oxygen tank."

"Okay, Ma," was all I said, but this was very upsetting for me on the inside. She didn't think of the dangers of the altitude before she headed for the hills, as if there was nothing to be concerned about. She had lived in Colorado for over ten years and was certainly familiar with the decreased oxygen level at higher altitudes and any danger that resulted from that. At least she used to be aware of this, whereas now it appeared to be a non-issue. Things worked out on this occasion, but it raised yet another red flag of concern for me.

Right after this I thought, "So this is what they mean by being a member of the sandwich generation." Between raising and worrying about my fifteen and eleven-year-old daughters, I was also caring for, and worrying about, my independent, car-gunning, renegade mother with decision-making issues. Apparently, without previously knowing it, and through no conscious action on my part, I was now a confirmed member of Club Sandwich. As a member of this club I kept a closer and closer eye on my mom because her incidents were becoming more frequent. From driving, to contact with strangers, to problems in her house, the issues continued. It was only a matter of time before she began to have issues within her own family.

MARY ANN

Enter my sister, Mary Ann. In December 2008, she received her doctorate in the nursing field. She was a teacher at a private university in the Chicago area and the mother of four grown kids. In May 2009, an aneurysm burst in her brain and she's never been remotely the same. She was in ICU, unconscious, for months. Eventually she regained consciousness, but she has been mentally and physically handicapped ever since and needs around the clock care. It was a devastating event on many levels, for her and her family, as well as for those of us in her extended group of family and friends.

When this happened, my mom had a very difficult time with it and understandably so. We all deal with tragedy in our own way, that's for sure, and Ma dealt with this in her own way. After she started to show the early signs of dementia, she'd sometimes yell at Mary Ann on the phone. Sometimes during this period, when I was at Ma's house, the answering machine would pick up the phone call and we'd hear Mary Ann talking and Ma would say, "Shhhh, don't answer the phone."

"Ma, why don't you answer the phone, it's Mary Ann?"

"I don't want to because all she wants to do is talk about Dad and ask if he's dead. I've told her a bunch of times that he was dead, but she always forgets and asks me again."

I said, "But Ma, she does that with everybody. She'll sometimes ask if Dad's alive three or four times in the same conversation. You just have to be patient with her and answer her questions."

"No!"

She just had a heck of a time dealing with Mary Ann's situation. In her defense, I can't imagine how hard this would be for a parent (or a spouse or a child, either) to deal with. Put this on top of the fact that Ma started showing the early signs of dementia a few years after Mary Ann's aneurysm, and this led to the behavior that I mentioned above. Brain trauma is not to be taken lightly.

Ma frequently went to Chicago to visit family and friends. On one of her trips she was at Mary Ann's house and she became so upset with Mary Ann's questions that she slammed her hand on the counter top and screamed at Mary Ann that, "Yes, your father is dead! One of these days I'm going to drive you out to the cemetery and show you his grave and then you'll know he's dead!"

Mary Ann was crying. Some of the other people present were crying. Ma seemed oblivious to this and when I asked her why she had to slam her hand and yell she said, "Because I wanted to make her understand that her dad was dead."

This was NOT my mom. She hadn't received the dementia diagnosis yet (this was in early 2013), but we were surely seeing more and more signs. I suppose, in her state, that this type of behavior was acceptable. Mary Ann's immediate family decided that Ma shouldn't be at their house for a bit, until they invited her when the time was right, because it was too upsetting for Mary Ann. I asked her about it again later, and she said she had no recollection of anyone telling her that she couldn't go to Mary Ann's house without an invitation.

In the summer of 2013, Ma made her last trip to Chicago. It was very hot, and my brother Jim said that when she got out of the car at his house, she looked like she was almost dead. She was overheated, dehydrated, white as a sheet, and stumbling. She didn't remember how to use the air conditioning in her car, so things got a little toasty. Jim asked her why she hadn't asked somebody at a gas station about the air conditioning and she said it wasn't necessary and that she was fine. Sure. She'd ask a stranger to plunge out her toilet, but she wouldn't ask for help with maintaining a reasonable core temperature. In her mind, these were all acceptable things to do, but it was far removed from her normal self and very alarming for the rest of us.

Jim and I both reminded her that she shouldn't just pop in at Mary Ann's and should wait until they invited her when the timing was right for Mary Ann. This had no effect on her actions and she showed up at Mary Ann's the next day, early. This was upsetting for the entire household and poor Ma was so confused about the whole thing. She spent a couple more days with Jim and his family and then zipped back home to Colorado.

ALL DOWNHILL FROM HERE

MID-SEPTEMBER 2013

Almost every fall I go on a fishing trip to the Ozarks. After the trip this year, the day I returned home was the same day that my mom was heading to California to see Bill, although she left several hours before I arrived. I had been in touch with Sandy on the phone while I was gone and, as expected, Ma was completely freaked out about making the trip. She was going to take the train, which required her to take a bus from Colorado Springs to Raton, New Mexico, where she'd board the train for Los Angeles. After she arrived in Los Angeles, she then planned to take a bus from the train station to Bill's town, just north of L.A. The night before the trip Ma stayed at our house because it seemed to her that this would make things easier for everybody. It didn't, but she thought it would. That evening, Sandy was cleaning up the supper dishes and when she turned around Ma was in a chair and had her head down on the kitchen table. She asked, "What's wrong, Nancy?"

"I don't know," Ma said.

"Are you nervous about going on this trip?"

"I don't know," Ma said. She was a nervous wreck.

The plan was for everyone to get up at six a.m. and get her to the bus station by seven, which was easily doable. At five a.m., Ma decided that Sandy and the kids had slept long enough so she rounded them up and away they went. They were at the bus station before six and then had to wait in the parking lot until seven for the bus. Sandy and the kids stayed to make sure Ma boarded okay. As she was going up the bus stairs my youngest daughter said, "Gramma's going on the bus, but it looks like she should be going to the hospital."

She made it to L.A. but the trip, once again, almost did her in. Shortly after getting off the train she knew that she needed to find the correct bus to Bill's, but she wasn't able to do it. Eventually, she reached the point where she couldn't even call Bill and instead she handed her phone to a train station employee and asked for their help. The kind man she handed her phone to called Bill and explained the situation. Bill then drove down to the train station and picked Ma up and brought her back to his place. And once again, Bill had to drive her home because she just wasn't in any condition to sit on a train and bus by herself for the long trip from Los Angeles to Colorado Springs. She was out of sorts for several days after that but slowly she somewhat returned to near-normal. Unbeknownst to all of us at the time, this was the last trip she would ever take by herself.

THE SANEST PERSON AROUND

Ma called me at work in early October 2013 and said that she just felt like crying and was very sad. She felt like she was "Going crazy or something."

This caught me completely off guard and gave me quite a scare. She sometimes called me when I was at work but never with this type of news. I called Sandy, who was home that day, and she went over to my mom's house and took her to the primary care doctor who then started the process to admit her to the mental hospital. The hospital's real name was a nice sounding euphemism, but it was a mental hospital all the same. None of us had ever been in one before, so it was a learning experience for all concerned. Spending time there was sure an eye-opener and a surreal experience for her, as well as for me. I am so grateful for the hospitals, other medical care facilities, and their wonderful employees. It takes a special kind of person to be a medical caregiver and, even though these places seem to be somewhat disorganized and a general pain in the butt, they are surely a godsend when needed.

Sandy brought Ma to the hospital and I came up shortly afterwards and saw her through the admission process. She went to the safest section, which was nice. I'm sure there were some areas in the facility that could have been somewhat dangerous due to aggressive, or possibly violent, patients.

I went to see her the next night after work and she didn't know why she was in there. She whispered to me, "I'm the sanest person in this place."

I said, "Ma, I checked with three other patients on the way in and they all told me that THEY were the sanest person in this place."

This met with no response. As far back as I can remember my mom had a great sense of humor, mixed in with sarcasm when the occasion called for it. It was a family trait - her siblings and their spouses were the same way. Jokers across the board. But now her sense of humor was fading away, at least for the time being. Either that or the joke wasn't that funny.

We talked about how she was feeling. I asked her what she did that day and she said, "Nothin'."

She was supposed to meet with a therapist, but it had not happened yet. I checked with the nurse and she checked her notes and confirmed that Ma actually had done "nothin' " that day. Every couple of days I'd go see her and she eventually met with a therapist that administered various psychological evaluation tests. Ma mentioned that the place was very disorganized.

Shortly after her admittance to the hospital, I went over to her house and went through her drawers, cabinets, and closets. She told me that she had a little cash hidden, so I removed that, and any other valuables, from her house for safekeeping. As I went through her dresser drawers, I found a couple dinner plates and bowls. Oooops, how'd they get in there? In the next drawer down, I found three complete newspapers. They weren't commemorative newspapers, just your standard, run of the mill daily papers, crammed into the drawer.

Her house had always been picked up, not white glove clean, but generally organized. At this point, it was a mess. I was at her house on a regular basis, but not in her bedroom drawers and closets so finding the house like this shook me up a bit. One part of me felt that she was going to be fine after some counseling, and maybe some medication, while she was in the hospital. Another part of me wondered why, back at her house, there were notes everywhere. I found four notes on the kitchen table and each one contained my phone number. Now, this was a woman who could quickly recite the alphabet backwards when she was seventy-seven years old. Really. She had a knack for remembering ten-digit phone numbers. Apparently, she was worried about forgetting mine, which made sense, but finding these notes made me sad. Very, very sad. I tried to remain stoic and act like all was well and that this was just a temporary setback.

As the days went on, she had several sit-down sessions with her counselor and doctor. The nursing staff was also evaluating her. One day her counselor called me and explained that the tests she had taken indicated that she had vascular dementia.

Finally. We finally had a proper diagnosis.

I had known things weren't right with her for some time, but now it was official. The counselor informed me that Ma would most likely need to go to assisted living upon her release. During her stay, Ma always made it a point to let me know that, "This place isn't very organized. I never see any doctors. I don't even know why I'm in here."

One evening, after my visit to the hospital, I was on the phone with my brother Jim, telling him about my visit to the hospital. Right in the middle of our conversation I had an epiphany that we'd done everything we possibly could, to keep her as independent as we possibly could, for as long as possible, and there had been no car accidents or serious injuries because of her living alone. This was a profound thought for me and helped me greatly with further decision making. This was the sign I'd been waiting for – it was time to take her car keys away. As much as it hurt me to do so, her driving days were over.

On her next to the last day in the mental hospital, Ma was to receive neuro-psych tests by yet another doctor. I asked the counselor if these tests could have any effect on changing my mom's diagnosis. She informed me that there was no way that the tests could do anything like that.

When the discharge date arrived, Sandy and I were there to pick her up. Approximately one hour before her checkout time, Sandy and I had an exit interview with the counselor and she told us, "The results from the neuro-psych test yesterday show that your mom does indeed have dementia, but she is still capable of making her own decisions."

"Wait a minute," I said, "now she can make her own decisions? I thought she was heading for assisted living. I've been calling people all over the place telling them this and now, in effect, you're telling me that instead of assisted living she can jump in her car, RIGHT NOW, and drive through the night to Tijuana! I thought you said that the tests wouldn't change anything?"

She said, "Well, sometimes doctors disagree."

I came back with, "That's fine if you're talking about the best way to treat an ear infection, but now I'm hearing that there's been a complete reversal of the initial decision."

"Yes," she said, "yes, that's right."

Somehow, it was possible for an off-site psychiatrist to overrule the resident head of the psych department at the hospital. This all seemed so very odd to me. I never met, or heard from, any of the doctors about any of this. I understand that doctors are busy, but come on. They'd RECOMMEND assisted living. They'd RECOMMEND drivers training and evaluation for the elderly. In the doctor's defense, maybe it isn't their place to help with these kinds of decisions. Maybe they specifically avoid this, and similar topics, because they feel it's best for the patient's family to decide. Perhaps they don't want the responsibility of taking away the patient's independence. Yet they seemed willing to let them continue to drive and possibly hurt themselves or others by not mandating a driving test. And, in our case anyway, Mom's doctor disregarded the report from the driver's test. It cost many thousands of dollars to stay in the hospital, but then she didn't receive much definitive help when it came to post-discharge matters. It seemed like I had to be the one to make the big decisions, without much help from any of the doctors. Maybe that's how it's supposed to be, I don't know. I'm sure that they can justify their positions, and I was certainly a rookie on this particular playing field, but I did feel a bit let down.

After her discharge, Ma stayed with us at our house and, two nights later around bedtime, she couldn't figure out which way to go from the entryway to her bedroom, which was less than ten feet away. Oh yeah, she can make her own decisions all right. Perhaps the neuro psych tests were a bit inconclusive? They were certainly not the do-all-end-all because, if I hadn't been watching her closely, she could have easily wandered out my front door in her nightgown, and ended up strolling around bewildered, on top of the mesa on the edge of the Rocky Mountain foothills, in the company of coyotes, bobcats, and the occasional mountain lion.

While staying with my family and me during this period, Ma made the comment several times that, "All these issues are new to me."

I gently explained to her that she was the only one who felt that this was new behavior. Sandy, Jim, Tom, the grandkids, and Aunt Mary, among others, had known about this for some time. It was only new to her. This confused her greatly, but she didn't bring it up again. It's worthwhile noting that she had the awareness to realize that something wasn't right. It was as if her normal brain was engaging in a tug-of-war with dementia, and dementia was winning. And drawing her into the quicksand.

During this time, Ma and I had several talks about her not driving. I told her I wouldn't let her drive anymore. "But I still want to be ABLE to drive," she said.

"Uh, what?"

"I just want to be able to drive in case Bill and I are out somewhere, and he needs me to drive."

"Okay, Ma. Sure. In that situation, of course you can drive."

"And I want to be able to drive to the doctor."

"I can drive you to the doctor, Ma."

She didn't like that answer one bit but backed off for the time being. She was fighting it with everything she had. Although never a physically strong person, she did possess a strong and, when necessary, stubborn mind. It was admirable, but sometimes it was difficult for me to keep calm during these episodes because I seem to have inherited these same traits. I had to let it go and do my best not to enter into an argument with her. You can't push an agenda based on logic, where little, or no, logic exists.

We also discussed moving her into an Assisted Living Facility (ALF). Sometimes she said that was fine. Other times she'd say she wanted to live alone in her house. She was quite confused with just about everything. Her decline was so rapid that, in my layman's mind it seemed that maybe she'd had a stroke or something similar. This wasn't likely though, because when she was in the hospital they'd checked her out and this wasn't the case.

As the days went on, Ma increasingly began to fight against the idea of going to assisted living. She insisted that she could stay at her own house if we'd just have somebody check on her a couple times a day. We didn't think it was a good idea but decided to give it a test run and see how it went. A few days later, Sandy dropped Ma off at her own house at eight thirty a.m. A friend of ours was a caregiver and experienced in such matters so she went over and joined Ma for a couple hours in the morning. Ma spoke to her several times, about how she needed to get stuff out of the house and get it sold. My translation was that she was not comfortable living alone. She was scared, and that scared me. I can't recall many times in my life when I'd seen her outwardly frightened. Maybe she just hid it well or maybe she really wasn't easily spooked.

In the summer of 1970, when I turned eleven years old, we took a family vacation to Alaska. All six of us packed into Dad's green Chevy pickup, with a camper on the back (a cab-over camper). My siblings ranged in age from seven to twelve. We headed north into Wisconsin, then Minnesota, and then over the border into Canada. From there we headed west, aiming for the Alaskan Highway. At one point, we were driving through the forest on a desolate dirt road, in the rainy mist and mud. I was quite young, so I don't remember the fine details, but suddenly there was something wrong with the truck. Maybe we were out of gas. Whatever the problem was, we were stranded, and my mom and dad made the decision that Dad would stay in the camper with us four kids and Ma would walk for help. That had to have been an extremely difficult decision for both of them to make.

One thing I remember vividly was looking out the window of the camper, watching my mom walk away in jeans and a gray hoodie, alone, into the drizzly fog. Nancy the Brave headed out by herself and came back with help. I don't remember what happened after that, but I'm here writing this so, apparently, everything worked out. Many years later Ma and I were talking about this trip and when we talked about the stranded truck episode, she told me that she had been scared to death, especially when she turned around and couldn't see the truck anymore. Our mom, our hero.

Sandy picked Ma up from her house in the early evening and brought her back to our house. I got home from work and talked with her and she was generally okay, but around eight p.m. she started to get down in the dumps. Generally, she liked to stay up until ten or ten thirty, but this night she went to her room a little after nine. I checked on her and she said that she had nothing else to do. I ask her what she wanted to do, and she replied, "I'm fine."

I figured she was just exhausted.

SOS - 10/15/2013

My alarm went off at four a.m. the next morning and I was exercising the snooze button, trying to get motivated. I'm a field engineer in the high-tech industry and work a twelve-hour shift. Having long weekends is nice, but the long work days get rougher with each passing year and this one was no exception.

I heard Ma get up and then heard the toilet flush. I finally crawled out of bed at four thirty and went to the kitchen. It was pitch black except for the front porch light shining through the glass in the front door. Suddenly, I saw a flashing light coming from the couch in the corner of the living room. It was flashing on and off like an SOS signal. Like Morse code. Huh?

I went over by the couch and there was my mom, somewhat curled up in the fetal position and holding a flashlight in her hand. She was crying and shaking. Trembling might be a better word. For a moment, I was stunned and couldn't talk. I sat on the edge of the couch, by her head, and wrapped my arms around her the best I could under the circumstances, "What's wrong, Ma?"

Through her sobs she said, "I don't know. I'm scared to death of everything. It's very bad and I'm afraid of hurting myself with knives and scissors."

I thought she was talking about hurting herself with knives or scissors when she tried to open her boxes of medicine patches that she had to wear every day. As she went on, I found out I was wrong. She said, "I've had thoughts of doing myself in so that the pain would stop."

Whoa! Stop right there. My mom was talking about killing herself. It seemed to me like she needed to go back to the hospital for further evaluation. Didn't they just recently decide that she was capable of making her own decisions? I left the room for a minute and told Sandy what was going on. She got up and made Ma a cup of tea and was consoling her on the couch while Ma quietly talked non-stop, slowly rocking from side to side. Sandy had positioned the couch in the middle of the living room floor so that Ma could look at the fire in the fireplace. I approached the couch from the rear and just seeing my mom slowly rocking and talking like this, I lost it. I couldn't stop the tears, so I quickly left the room before they knew I was there. No reason to upset Ma more than she already was. I went into the bathroom at the other end of the house and splashed cold water on my face several times, doing my best to regain a little composure.

The kids were up by then, due to all the commotion, and they were kinda freaked out. They knew that gramma had not been right, but this was a completely new level of "not right." Ma continued with her talking and sometimes she'd just start sobbing again and was, to my untrained eyes, having some sort of breakdown. She'd say things like, "Just stick me somewhere, I'll be fine."

She then wanted me to call Bill and let him know that she had "flipped her lid." On one hand, she was having, or had just had, a serious mental episode. On the other, she was cognizant of the fact that something wasn't right, yet she was still able to somewhat make a joke about it. She was also very concerned about disturbing our household. As I studied her face, she truly looked mentally ill. Her eyes were sunken and the skin around her eyes was darkish. The rest of her face was quite white, almost ashen. She trembled when she spoke and was obviously weak.

After a few hours we were able to contact her primary care doctor, and then back to the mental hospital we went. This time I knew right where to park, who to talk to, and how to get the ball rolling. I explained to the staff that although she had not acted suicidal, she had certainly made suicidal comments. They took all this down during the admission process and then they wheeled her away, back to the area where she had just been released from the week before.

A few days later, I received a call from the head doctor (finally!) and she explained that the vascular dementia that Ma had been diagnosed with was most likely the result of her long-term high blood pressure. This struck me as a little strange because she'd been on medication to control her high blood pressure for decades and I didn't understand how controlled high blood pressure could be the cause? The doctor then explained how high blood pressure could cause hardening of the arteries, which can then lead to vascular dementia. Apparently, hardening of the arteries can also sometimes lead to a TIA (Transient Ischemic Attack – sometimes called a mini-stroke). In addition, hardening of the arteries can also lead to random memory loss and mood swings, among other problems. To top it all off, the lack of vascularity to her brain, due to the hardened arteries, was causing her brain to shrink.

The doctor continued with the fact that Ma needed to be in assisted living due to sundowning, as well as for medication control. I assumed that there'd be some mention of her depression and suicidal thoughts, but that never came up. Later that night I talked to the kids and tried to smooth things over for them a little bit. I explained how their grandma was sick, confused, and afraid of many things. I told them how this wasn't her fault and we just needed to love her and help her as much as we could.

The next day, Sandy and I visited a few assisted living facilities after calling around and trimming our options down to three. The first one was a four-plex that the owners converted to an assisted living unit and was designed like a house. There was a kitchen and central common area with couches and a TV. Then there were four bedrooms, one for each of the residents. On site there was a full time CNA to do the cooking and take care of the residents. It was a different kind of concept that I knew my mom wouldn't be comfortable with at all, so we crossed it off the list.

The next place was a lower-end facility and we didn't like the feel of it, either. In general it was okay, and we liked the staff that we talked to, but it had several things I didn't like. There was no carpet anywhere. The dining area was filled with long white tables and hard plastic chairs, similar to a grade school cafeteria. It was cold and uncomfortable. The rooms were all two-person rooms and very small with no closet, just a wall locker. There was very little privacy anywhere. It certainly would have worked if necessary, but at that time it wasn't necessary, so we crossed it off the list as well.

It's worth mentioning that both places smelled like urine. Now, sometimes people become incontinent, especially in these types of settings, but just the smell turns me off right away (this is not to imply that some people enjoy this smell, right away). If I'm sitting in a soft, comfortable chair in the lobby, and I smell urine, it's like the chair I'm sitting in had urine on it at some point. The same thing goes for a rug or couch or, well, you get the idea. I have a big nose and don't miss much in the smell department and I was not going to have my mom stay in a place that reeked of urine.

We eventually made it over to the third facility that we had pre-selected and, to be perfectly honest with you, I could still smell urine in the car and in the parking lot because it was still in my nose hairs or whatever. It's also worth mentioning that neither Sandy nor I smelled like urine (other than my nose hairs). When we entered the third facility there were automatic doors that opened as we walked up from the parking lot. And when they opened, it was like entering Shangri La. The nicely carpeted floors led up to nicely decorated walls that gave the place an overall warm feeling. There was a lovely smell of fragrant candles (none of which smelled like urine) and there was a beautiful dining area, reading area, and a separate library. A huge fish aquarium graced one wall and there was a separate area for exercise classes and the like. We heard soft piano music playing over the sound system and further exploration revealed that the sound was actually someone PLAYING a piano in an area that had initially been out of our line-of-sight. We received the grand tour and liked what we saw very much. All the rooms were private rooms with walk-in closets and a private bathroom. And to top it all off, the overall cost was less expensive than the previous two places we'd visited. This was to be my mom's new home.

The next night, I visited Ma in the hospital. She was clear and sharp, and, at face value, she appeared to be her old self. She got my jokes and understood when I was teasing her. She even teased me back a little. She was very lucid, and I came close to asking myself, "What's she doing in here?" In retrospect, I should have been more aware of these lucid moments of hers. I should have capitalized on them and spent even more time with her when they occurred. It's not as if I was in complete denial, I just wasn't fully aware of the long-term nature of her condition. While she was in this state, I asked her several financial type questions concerning her household finances and she was right on top of things. It was hard to believe that she had been crying uncontrollably on my couch the day before.

The next day, Ma was back to being cranky. She frequently talked about the other patients, sometimes even when they were right next to us, or otherwise well within earshot. She'd say loudly, "I'm not sure what's wrong with this guy!"

"This guy over here shakes really bad and I don't know what's wrong with him!"

She made no effort to keep her voice down, which was a noticeable change from her pre-dementia state. She had always been lively for the most part, but she was not overly outgoing and wouldn't do anything to call attention to herself. Commenting on some of the other patients was something she might have previously done under her breath, but the audible commentary was a sad sign that she was becoming a different person. Her personality was eroding before my eyes, and there was nothing I, or anyone else, could do to stop it.

A couple days later found her still cranky and mildly depressed. "There's something just not right about this place," she said. She asked why she couldn't go home, and I told her that it was much better for her to move into assisted living because, among other things, I couldn't have her talking about suicide in front of the kids. She said, "That's life," implying that the kids should be able to hear these kinds of things because, "that's life."

She didn't say it nicely, or in any kind of light-hearted manner. She said it as a statement of fact. Holy cow, where'd my mom go?

Sandy and the kids frequently visited grandma in the hospital. Ma told Sandy the same story about living with us, or at her house with a caregiver checking on her daily. She was desperately trying to change her inner situation by changing her outer circumstances. It was all she knew how to do. She pronounced that she didn't want, or need, anti-depressants, because she was the most non-depressed person you could find.

During one of my visits, I noticed that she was looking a bit disheveled. It turned out she hadn't taken a shower since her admittance to the hospital six days prior because she didn't feel safe and was uncomfortable showering there. I persuaded her to take a shower, and I guarded the perimeter while she did so. She still hadn't received any anti-depressants. This was also the day when the head nurse from the Assisted Living Facility (ALF) came to the hospital and did an assessment on Ma as a prerequisite to her upcoming admittance to the ALF.

I had several questions for Ma about her finances again because I was still getting her affairs in order. She was okay, but her mental health was down several steps from prior to the California trip. It seemed like several years earlier but, in reality, it had only been a month. She also didn't remember many aspects of her basic financial information – but she did know some of it. This was a much different response than the one I heard from her when we discussed finances five days prior. She still wanted to be able to drive, but "just to the doctor."

A friend of mine had a mother with dementia at this same time and she tried the exact same "just to the doctor" angle with him. How can this be? Is it possible that there's one deceptive neural pathway left when a person is in the throes of dementia, which results in them trying to hang on to their car keys by saying that they want to be able to drive, "just to the doctor?" Maybe.

After one week, I still couldn't get a doctor to return my calls. I had several questions concerning my mom's situation that I wanted to discuss prior to her discharge. The therapist called, but she was new at this and, although very nice, somewhat clueless. She told us that Ma had to evacuate the premises at ten a.m. the next day. I asked for one more day, due to my work schedule, to get my mom's assisted living room squared away. I planned to move her stuff in the next day, Wednesday, and Ma in on Thursday, but they couldn't let her stay one extra night due to hospital rules, which meant she'd be spending the night with us.

Sandy contacted me early in the day and said that the ALF called and told her that they'd assessed my mom as a Care Level three. What!? FYI - level one was $525/month, level two was $775/month and level three was $1025! This was, of course, in addition to the price for the room every month.

When talking to the ALF early in the process, they asked me if Ma could feed herself. Yes. Wash herself? Yes. Dress herself? Oh yeah. Walk unassisted? Yes. That sounded like a level one to the person I talked to – minimal care needed other than medication control and generally keeping an eye on her. But now, the head ALF nurse assessed Ma in the mental hospital and found out from the nurses there that Ma had been "restless" at night. She tended to wander and say, "I want to go home."

Incidentally, we never heard ONE WORD about this from anyone at the hospital. The point here is that if she was wandering around when in the ALF, then it would require extra staff time to round her up and put her back in her room, which is why she was assessed as a level three. We then found out that, while in the hospital, they had increased her dementia medication to the full-dose amount. Now they were going to adjust it back down to the half-dose amount, just prior to her discharge, because the full dose caused her to become agitated!

In summary, the hospital upped her medication, which was standard procedure for this medication, and it made her agitated and restless. Then, the head nurse from the ALF assessed her and raised her up to a level three, because at night she was, uh, restless. No biggie, it'd just cost another $500/month (cynicism intended).

I explained to the ALF head nurse that as far as I knew, Ma never wandered at night before the mental hospital and that level three seemed excessive to me. She finally relented and dropped it down to a level two which, somehow, was supposed to make me feel better as it was only $250/month higher than level one. She stated that they would reassess Ma after thirty days and at that time we'd see what level they could change her to, if necessary. I then asked her whom I could call once a week to check and see if my mom was wandering at night. That way I could nip it in the bud with her primary care doctor and get her meds adjusted. She assured me that I did not need to call because if something wasn't right in the Mom department, they'd contact me ASAP.

Released on 10/23/2013

They released Ma from the hospital and, near as I could tell, they did absolutely NOTHING to address her depression issues or her suicidal thoughts. Perhaps they felt that the depression was due to the dementia, but they never did expound on it any further. I brought her to our house for the night and she was very agitated and "just wanted to live with us."

She was intermittently crying and mentally down. She wanted to stay at her house with a caregiver checking on her. She wanted to drive. My kids were upset. Before I got home with Ma, my oldest daughter climbed up the tree in the front yard and stayed there for a while, to avoid gramma's unpredictable behavior. When we first got home, I set Ma up in the front room and turned the TV on for her. A little while later I went in and checked on her. She was kinda nodding off, so I tickled her behind the ear and she about jumped out of her skin. This was VERY upsetting to her. She let out a short exclamation but was unable to talk. If looks could kill, it would've been the end of me. I felt like an idiot when all I was trying to do was loosen her up. I had noticed over the last year that if anything or anyone startled her in any way, it was a very traumatic experience. Unfortunately for both of us, I had forgotten about this at the time of the ear tickle.

That evening, we were sitting at the dining room table and she was much calmer than she had been earlier. I talked to her quite a bit about the changes she was going through, and she was openly talking about it. This was somewhat unusual for her, but welcome. She was from the school of "Everything's fine. I'll be all right. Don't worry about me."

Although she didn't always care for small talk, and it certainly wasn't unusual for her to be on the shy side in the past we, nonetheless, had many, many lengthy conversations over the years. And tonight was starting out to be one of those times. She was quite pensive at first and said, "Well, there are a lot of things for me to do when I move into my new room. And the place is nice."

"Sure Ma, they have all kinds of activities for you there, so you should be able to stay busy."

"There's even a piano so maybe I can start playing again," she said. "And there's lots of places where I can walk, too."

"That's right Ma, and I'll be over there to visit you a lot and Sandy and the kids will come regularly too, and we'll also come get you and bring you over to our house, so you can spend time away occasionally."

"Oh that'd be just great," she said as she perked up even further, "and Bill can come visit me and we can travel around taking photos."

She was open to many of these ideas and her eyes were not as sad as they had been recently. They weren't quite sparkling, but they were certainly lit up a bit. She had a bit of hope in her voice along with a closer-to-normal skin tone. It was refreshing for me as well, refreshing to still see glimpses of the Mom that I had always known.

I explained that I was doing my best to get her situation squared away, and to find a nice place for her to live, which calmed her down a bit more. But then she became quite upset about not being able to control her own medications. "I'm quite capable of taking my own medications," she said in a louder voice. "And I'm starting to feel trapped!" she yelled.

I told her it was easy for me to understand why she'd feel that way. Her pensive mood was turning darker and her eyes started to moisten as her frustration mounted. Then she instantly calmed down and in a very sad and quiet voice said, "I'm starting to lose control of my life."

I explained that in some ways she was losing control of her life, but that it was for the best because we had to make sure that she was in a safe place. Without another word she slowly got up from the table and started to shuffle out of the room. Her energy had drained away and it took everything she had just to walk the short distance to the bedroom. Her head was down and, although I couldn't see her eyes, I could tell that she was crying. I put my arms around her, stopping her in her tracks, and kissed her on top of the head and said, "I know that all this stinks, Ma, and I wish we didn't have to do it, but I really am doing what I think is best for you."

"I know you are honey," she said, as we walked into the bedroom and I tucked her in for the night.

It dawned on me that night that we had been charged $200 more than we had agreed upon for the room at the ALF. When I signed the contract for her residency earlier in the day, I found out that the prices typically went up six to ten percent a year, but usually six. We'll see. Then I discovered the $200 overcharge. It looked like the cost had gone up 6.5% already and she wasn't even living there yet.

MOVE-IN DAY - 10/24/13

As we were driving over to the ALF with Ma for the first time, she couldn't figure out where we were in town. It was about ten minutes from my house, but she had no idea where we were. In addition, this was the day when she started saying "okay."

I mean she REALLY started saying "okay."

Now, we all say okay occasionally, don't we? That's not what I'm talking about here. This was another sign that she was continually becoming a different person. I think she said okay so often because she couldn't think of anything else to say. It was as if, under certain circumstances, she knew that she wanted to say something as part of what we'd consider a normal conversation, but she couldn't come up with anything other than "okay." We were driving in the car, and the kids were in the back seat. Ma was sitting in the passenger seat and whenever there was a lull in our talking and she couldn't think of a topic, she started to chant, "Okay……O..kay……Okay." She was so very nervous, out of sorts, and confused with what was going on. It upset me and must've been horrible for her.

She also started another new habit that day as we drove over to the ALF. She felt it was necessary to begin reciting the name on any street sign she'd see, or any business sign on a building or on the side of a truck, or whatever else she saw. As we were driving down the street, any street, she'd let it rip, "BDE engineering…what's that other word… Con..Con consultants, okay."

I took her over to her house, first, so that she could pick up a few things. On the way over to the ALF from there, she read every street sign and business sign that she could. "Oh, there's Swope, the street where you used to live. Let's go take a ride down there and see how your old house looks."

A few minutes later "Oh! There's Custer Street. That's where Jenny lives. She's so pretty, and nice too! I wonder how she's doing?"

Sometimes, if I knew we were coming upon a street sign with an exceptionally long name, I'd slow down so she had time to read it all. As we approached the ALF, I pointed out the main street in front of her building, several times. I showed her the big park across the street. The kids and I walked around the grounds with her, three times. She was, understandably, shell-shocked.

I took her up to her private room. "The room is small," she said.

Several of the staff came by to visit while we were in her room and they were all very nice. Ma was upset but generally took things in stride. We went back down to the restaurant for lunch and as we were finishing, the head of the dining services came out and talked with her. He was a very friendly guy and, before long, I whispered to him that we were going to sever the ties right away. I motioned to the kids to head out (they had already hugged gramma). I gave her a hug, kissed her head and said, "I love you, Ma. We'll leave you talking with your new friend."

She wanted, and of course received, one more hug. Then we left, which was very hard to do because I wanted to stay. It was not unlike leaving your child on their very first day of school. It was for the best, but I still felt like I was abandoning her.

PLAYING WITH A FULL DECK?

The next day, the kids and I went to Ma's house and picked up her TV and some medications she had there and then brought them over to the ALF. I explained to the kids that I was very concerned about how gramma would adjust to her new surroundings. We were carrying items in the front door, and there was Ma. I spotted her right away, with her back to us on a couch and participating in the current exercise class. Her head was dancing back and forth, and she was smiling from what I could see when she turned her head to the side. We didn't interrupt as we went up to her room with the TV and medicine. On the way we looked for, and found, the nurse's station. Then we encountered confusion from the staff as to where we should take the medicine we'd brought from my mom's house. After we straightened that out, we then went to Ma's room and waited for her exercise class to finish up. The kids and I were on the bed and I was very happy that Ma was exercising and smiling at the same time. A tear was beginning to form in the corner of my eye as I started to write a text to Sandy and my brothers about Ma's status, and how good things were looking after only one day. Then Ma burst into the room and said, "I don't belong here."

The teardrop dried up and never made it out. Then she went on about the meds. On her way to the room she had encountered a staff member in the hallway who cheerfully told her, "I have a pill for you."

Ma paused for effect, looked disgusted, threw up her hands and said, "Where's the pill?"

I told her that I knew exactly what she was trying to do about the meds and how, if she had been in charge, she would've had her pills squared away. I explained that, "You haven't even been here twenty-four hours and I just dropped the meds off fifteen minutes ago. Give 'em a chance, Ma." Within twenty minutes, a med tech arrived with her pills and that ended that conversation for the time being.

Ma previously mentioned that she wished she had a deck of cards. When I was at her house getting the TV that morning, I noticed an old deck of cards on the countertop. I explained to the kids that this would be a nice surprise for Gramma, and it would surely cheer her up! I had them in my pants pocket and forgot about them until she came into the room so, when she wasn't looking, I slid them on the desk.

I asked about her breakfast, lunch, and medications, although I was really trying to steer her attention to the desk. A few times, as she was wandering around the room, she'd come close to the desk but then turn away. I was on the edge of my seat because they were burning a hole in my mind and I couldn't wait to see her reaction. Eventually she spotted them, broke out with a big grin and asked, "Where did these come from? I've been looking for a deck of cards!"

I then explained that, "These are very old, and I didn't count the total number of cards, so I can't guarantee that you're playing with a full deck."

And she got the joke! She laughed harder and longer then I'd seen her do in quite some time. She even had to sit down until the spasms subsided. Mission accomplished.

I told her that Sandy would be there around five to pick her up and bring her over for supper. She said that she'd come downstairs to meet Sandy, but I said she should stay in her room because Sandy would want to see it. I explained, "Please wait for Sandy in your room and there's no need to worry if she's a couple minutes late. I promise she'll be here."

The kids and I headed home, and at five p.m. I received a phone call from the ALF. They explained that Ma had been in the lobby since four and was very nervous and confused as to why there was nobody there to pick her up. Sandy arrived a few minutes later and brought Ma over to our house where we all had supper and a few minutes after that Ma said she was tired and wanted to go home. Sandy and I took her home and went up to the room so that Sandy could check it out. When we arrived at her room, she and Sandy searched the hallways and found the laundry room, which was good because Ma said that she wanted to do her own laundry. I explained the phone situation to her, as I had done several times already, but it still confused her a bit. I then asked her if she wanted me to take the empty move-in boxes out of her room.

She said, "No, I'll need them for when I leave."

"You got it, Ma."

For weeks, she'd been VERY concerned about who was going to get what from her house. "People in Chicago may want my plants or clothes," she said.

She also wanted me to ask all her neighbors if they wanted any of her clothes. I told her that I did, but I really didn't.

That's because Tom's wife, Mai, loves a lot of Mom's clothes and I wanted to save them for her. To this day, my mom's Thai daughter-in-law can be seen in and around Chiang Mai in northern Thailand, wearing some of Mom's pants, blouses, and jewelry.

The next day was the first day we hadn't been with Ma since she moved in. I called her on her cell phone, and after a few minutes she said, "I feel like I'm going crazy and I'm afraid of everything. I want to go to the doctor and get a new brain."

She really said that – and meant it.

She wanted to live with my brother Jim, our sister Mary Ann, or me. She told me that she wouldn't do anything bad (?) and that she was feeling better. I told Jim, Tom, and Aunt Mary that if she continued to decline at this rate that it wouldn't be long before she didn't remember who we were and that I had no way of knowing how quickly the disease would progress.

I called Ma a couple days later to check on her and she said that, on Sunday morning, she only received one pill and it wasn't for blood pressure. I said, "Ma, give these people a chance to do their job because they do it every day and they're good at it, okay?"

I asked her about any pills she received Sunday night, but she couldn't remember. I told her I'd be there the next day and investigate it for her. She was very upset that she didn't have access to a pill that contained acetaminophen and a sleep aid, which she told me she'd been taking EVERY NIGHT for years. I explained that that sounded dangerous and she said, "Everybody I knows does it."

I told her that I didn't do it. My wife didn't do it. My two brothers didn't do it. In fact, I didn't know of anyone who did it, other than her. That didn't matter much, and she acted as if she hadn't heard a word I'd said. Later, in her house, I found her stash of several large bottles of these pills and threw them all away.

She then went on to tell me about the people that sat at her table in the dining room. There was one man, George, and his wife Mary Lou. She thought Mary Lou was nitpicky and didn't seem to like her husband George very much. I met Mary Lou a few days later and she was mentally in bad shape, but Ma couldn't see it. She told me that there was another woman who ate with her head down on the table, so Ma thought she was weird or crazy. It turned out that the poor woman had very advanced osteoporosis and wasn't capable of holding her head up by herself.

One evening I went to see Ma, and she was generally okay. I asked one of the med techs to come to the room, so I could talk to her about the pill situation. She said that my mom had only been getting one blood pressure med, and not the two that she should be getting. Excuse me? She also hadn't been getting the dementia patch or the anti-anxiety med. Excuse me? She said that it was because they had not received the doctor's orders yet. I told her that I'd call the doctor and get this resolved right away.

I figured that her blood pressure (BP) was probably under control seeing as she was still taking one BP medication. I wanted to check her BP with her own personal monitor, but the batteries were dead. I wrote a note for the night shift med tech and left the note with Ma and asked her to give it to the tech when she gave Ma her pills that evening. I went home and about 9:45 p.m. I received a call from the med tech and she asked me, "Do you know that your mom has not received ANY of her blood pressure meds since she's been here?"

Huh? That's five days. She also confirmed that Ma hadn't been receiving her dementia patch or anti-anxiety meds. She went on to say that the medicine I brought for Ma on Friday was not in the doctor's orders and that they needed to order the correct medication. The med tech gave this info to the nurse on shift and the nurse "blew it off."

Huh? Are you kidding? She apologized to me profusely and said this wasn't a very good first impression. She said she knew that we were kind, compassionate people but if it were her mom, she'd be calling tomorrow to let these people know how upset we were. I explained that this wouldn't be a problem and said, "Seeing as my mom hasn't been receiving her blood pressure meds, has anybody thought to check her blood pressure?"

Nope.

"Well, do you think we could get it checked RIGHT NOW?!"

She said she'd get right on it, and that she'd also contact the head nurse and see if she'd call me right then. I hung up and got ready to either take my mom to the hospital or take her old blood pressure meds that were still at my house, over to her. The tech called back and said that her blood pressure was 140/80, which was generally acceptable and certainly better than it could've been. She said that the head nurse would call me in the morning. This whole mess upset me so much that after I went to sleep, I woke up many times, wondering why they called this "assisted" living.

I was at work the next day and waiting for the head nurse to call. By ten a.m. she hadn't called, so I called and tracked her down. She said she was very sorry and would have a staff meeting and find out all the details and then call me back that afternoon. In the middle of the afternoon, she called back and provided me with the following info:

After we talked earlier that day, they ordered her correct blood pressure meds because of the initial mix-up. It turns out that a different nurse came on shift and saw the issue and took care of it. Therefore, Ma received her BP meds first thing in the morning. I asked if maybe they ordered the correct pills because of my phone call. She said, "No, it was due to the other nurse coming in and doing what needed to be done."

I tried not to think about how much I'd have to say after she'd been a resident for a month or two. At home afterwards, I came across a brochure for the ALF that I picked up when we first visited the place. It had a section that read, "We have promised ourselves that we will always treat our residents as we would our own loved ones. Only our best will do."

Right.

On Friday, Ma had an MRI appointment and I went to have breakfast with her beforehand. I told her on the phone that I'd meet her at her table, but she waited for me in the lobby anyway. I hugged her and apologized for having doubted her when she told me she was only getting one blood pressure pill. She said, "That's okay, honey."

The MRI was uneventful. Later, Sandy, the kids, and I all had supper with her at the ALF. Supper hours were from 4:30 - 6:00 but she insisted that we must be there at 4:30 and not one minute later. I saw, and then waved at, one of the med techs and she said, "Looks like we finally got those meds squared away!"

I was thinking, "And hey, at least she didn't have a carotid artery blow out the side of her neck."

The following day I took Ma to her primary care doctor and she had gained three pounds, which was huge for her. She was apparently eating regularly at the ALF and now weighed one hundred and twenty pounds. One hundred and thirty would probably have been better for her overall health and strength, but one-twenty was a good start. She asked the doc, "What am I gonna have to do to be able to go back home again? What do I have to prove to you?"

She was antsy and acted as if there was a glimmer of hope that her doctor would grant her an early release because he may have felt that crossing the one-hundred-and-twenty-pound barrier would do the trick. He handled it nicely and told her that first she'd have to be able to take care of herself. He then told her that she had stabilized nicely and that she was doing better. I then told her that the doctor wouldn't be the only one to make the decision as to when she went home again and that I'd be involved too, if I felt it was the safe thing to do. Then her heart sank, and she instantly stopped talking. This was so difficult for her to comprehend because she had always been such an independent person. It was eating her up inside as she struggled to understand what was happening, when a tear rolled down her left cheek. Then MY heart sank. Why did I have to say what I did? I just couldn't keep quiet about something that I knew was very important to her, even though I also knew darn well that she'd forget this entire episode in a short period of time. My knee-jerk reaction was totally uncalled for and I should have kept my comment to myself. I tried to maintain calm control when it came to these types of situations but I, apparently, still had a long way to go. Outwardly, I probably sounded like John the Drill Sergeant and that I was being entirely too controlling with her. This certainly wasn't my intent, but it pales in comparison to the internal beatings I frequently gave myself over my thoughtless comments. My mom wasn't the only one who was confused.

Later in the week, I went and picked Ma up and brought her back to our house for dinner. When I called and told her that I'd be over to pick her up she said, loudly, "Oh, you mean you're going to come and get me and bring me over to your house for dinner? That sounds wonderful!"

She said it as if I hadn't mentioned it to her before and that we'd never done anything remotely like it, ever. During supper, I also noticed for the first time that, in response to certain statements, she'd get this completely amazed and shocked look on her face. For example, at dinner one night my oldest daughter told her, "That's buffalo sauce, Gramma." Ma then grabbed the table with both hands, dramatically leaned back and had this look of utter astonishment on her face. As time went on, she responded in this manner to more and more events.

At the end of the day when I was dropping her off, I went into the lobby with her and she gave me her crumpled up, hand written, Christmas letter and asked me to edit it and type it up for her. For as long as I could remember, she'd write a letter like this to inform her family and friends of the happenings in her life near the end of the year. "Sure Ma, I'll type it up and then let you read it before we send them out. Sound good?"

She didn't answer. We were hugging at this point and she eventually said, "Please, please get me out of this place, honey. I'll do anything you want." She started crying as she clung to me and continued, "I can pay you and Sandy the same as it costs here at assisted living. I won't be any trouble, I promise."

Ouch. I didn't know what to do, or what to tell her. I kissed the top of her head and said, "I love you Ma." It was all I could think of doing at the time.

A few days later, I met with the ALF manager and spent two hours going over my perceived shortcomings of their operation. He acted like a true manager and told me what he thought I wanted to hear. He also promised to provide the documents that I requested. Mom called that evening and left a message asking me to please call the doctor and see when she would be able to go back to living at home again because she didn't want to live like this any longer.

I CAN'T FIND MY KEYS

11/8/2013 1:45:48 P.M.

Ma called and left a panicked message on my cell phone, and it sounded like she was crying, or on the verge, because she couldn't get into the locked cabinet in her room:

"Hi honey, I can't find my keys to get in the cabinet. I can't find my keys and I can't get in the cabinet to see if I put them in there. Can you please come down with that key? Oh, my God I'm trapped. Oh my God. And I can't go anywhere for another key because nobody would have it. Please call me and come with the key."

The cabinet she was talking about was a small, standard kitchen cabinet in her apartment that we had the maintenance guys put a small lock on, for her valuables and whatnot. It took a key to lock it and to open it. Therefore, there was no way she could have locked the keys inside the cabinet. She kept the key on an elastic wristband with her room key and mailbox key.

11/8/2013 1:48:39 P.M.

Not quite three minutes later there was another message:

"Hi honey. False alarm. I found my keys. They were on my wristband that slid way up on my shoulder and I couldn't feel them. I'm sorry. I hope you didn't leave already. I'm supposed to go out on my ride at two o'clock."

She was referring to her 'scenic ride' on the ALF shuttle bus, where residents could enjoy a scenic ride to various points of interest in and around Colorado Springs. Sometimes they'd go through Garden of the Gods park, a scenic area on the west edge of town, in the foothills and graced with numerous beautiful reddish-orange rock formations. Sometimes they'd go through the United States Air Force Academy, just north of Colorado Springs. On other trips they'd go through smaller parks in the area as well. Colorado Springs is a very beautiful city in spots and there's no shortage of destinations for sightseeing. After a while though, Ma complained that they kept going to the same spots over and over, which they did. Eventually, she didn't bring it up anymore because she forgot where they had gone in the past. And it wasn't long before she lost interest in going at all.

THE SPEECH

On this day, we had my oldest daughter's birthday party at our house. Sandy went to get Ma and when they arrived back at our house, Ma came back to my office where I was working at my desk. I gave her a copy of the end-of-year letter that she had previously asked me to edit and print for her. I asked her to read it and, if she liked it, I'd print out a bunch of copies so she could send them out. She said she wanted to use our house for the return address. I said that she should probably use her own address for the return address. She was quickly growing distraught and said, "I just don't want to live like that."

I said, "Ma, you're eating three meals a day, every day. You're participating in all kinds of activities and making new friends. If you were at home, you'd be sitting on the couch and looking out the window, wondering what to do with yourself."

I went on to explain the benefits of her current level of social interaction that she had not had consistently in twenty years. She said she just wanted somebody to come live at her house so that she could stay there. I asked, "Who are you going to get to live there, Ma?"

She was sad and said, "I don't know. Maybe if your brother Jim moves out here, one of his kids could live with me."

I said, "Ma, they're in their twenties, so even if they did move here they wouldn't be home very much."

I explained numerous times how it'd be best if she'd quit fighting her situation and just try to adapt to her new life, but she wouldn't have anything to do with it and I can't say that I would have responded any differently if I were in her shoes. What was readily apparent to me was incomprehensible to her; it wasn't even on her radar. This was my problem, not hers.

When the birthday party began, we walked out to the dining room for a late lunch and to join the fun. Right in the middle of the meal, my mom stood up, completely unannounced, without fanfare, and emotionally stated that, "This is really good food."

She was clearly emotional, trembling, choked up, and almost crying. Ten minutes later, completely unannounced, she rose up again and explained to everyone that, "I just want to thank John and Sandy for all they've done for me with my illness. If it wasn't for them, I don't know where I'd be right now."

This took the audience quite by surprise, but they rolled with it nicely. I must admit that I was speechless because this was so completely out of character for her that I didn't know how to act. In all the years that I'd known her, she never would have done anything remotely like this. Ever.

A few days later, in the morning, I went over to visit Ma. I went to the ALF sunroom while she finished up with her exercise class and then she came over to visit with me after the class was finished. I asked her how the workout went, and she said, in her most disgusted voice, "Twenty minutes late."

The woman at the front desk was walking around to stretch her legs and when Ma went to get a bottle of water the lady came over and told me that my mom usually helped people in the bingo room if they needed help reading the cards, or knowing where to put their markers on the card, and things like that. That was nice to hear. We went up to her room and I spotted an envelope on the nightstand, on which she had written, "If I'm alive, please don't open this."

She then mentioned that she found a new place to walk BEHIND SOME APARTMENT BUILDINGS. I explained that she shouldn't be walking there and should stay out in plain sight. Apparently, the adventurous part of her was still present but, equally apparent, was the fact that she was having trouble remembering basic safety precautions.

JOHN'S EPIPHANY

On the day when the ALF had their Thanksgiving buffet, Sandy, the kids, and I were there for the occasion. It was quite a spread to be sure and there were a couple hundred people present, residents and guests alike. The line at the buffet was quite long and resulted in a twenty-minute wait before getting to the food. Holiday music was playing in the background and the smell of cinnamon was in the air. We were all waiting in line, the place was in a festive mood, and we were talking with each other and several of the residents that we'd come to know.

After we'd been in line for ten minutes or so, I looked up and saw Paul, a new friend that I had talked with a few times, approaching us as he headed for the end of the line. He was a very gentle and soft-spoken man, tall and slightly hunched over. He wore glasses, jeans and, usually, a flannel shirt. I waved at him and he waved and then stopped when he reached me. We made small talk and I asked him if he'd like to cut in line with us and save some time. He looked around slowly, closely checking the length of the line behind us, thought about it, and softly said, "Might start a riot."

My laugh was uncontrollable! His timing was awesome, and it completely caught me off-guard. I must admit that, much earlier in my life, I assumed that all nursing home residents were lacking in their social skills. Obviously, this was a false assumption on my part, but I hadn't really thought about it again prior to my mom's diagnosis. I had no reason to. It was an outdated notion from my teen years when I worked at a nursing home and I hadn't been in this type of facility again since I was seventeen years old. Sure, some of the residents in these facilities were seriously suffering from dementia and the like, but not all of them. Thanks Paul.

When growing up in Oak Lawn, IL, I worked in the kitchen of a nursing home near 95th and Ridgeland. On one occasion, those of us in the kitchen crew were taking a break, seated at a large, round table in the resident's dining room. I had just started chewing on my last stick of gum and was minding my own business when an elderly woman rolled up to me in her wheelchair and asked me in her raspy voice, "Can I get a stick of that gum?"

I said, "I'm sorry, but it was my last piece."

She thought about this for a minute, looked me in the eye, and while rolling away said, "I hope you choke on it."

I was shocked! I didn't expect such a mean response from this woman who reminded me of my grandmother. Now, she may have been mean from day one, but it may also have been a case like my mom's where the angriness was one of the many symptoms of her illness.

The next week, Ma mentioned that she had received a scratch-type sweepstakes ticket in the mail. She scratched it and found out that she had four kings. She called me up and really wanted me to check it out because the chances of having four kings were one in TEN MILLION. The prize was ten thousand dollars. She said that she really wanted to win this, because at least then she'd be able to leave her kids something, seeing as how the assisted living place was taking all her money.

The following day, she called again and said she'd leave the card lying on her bed so that I could come right over and check it out while she was gone. When I finally checked the card, I discovered that recipients "might be subjected to a demonstration" of some sort. It was an advertisement for an air purification system. I read further that, for any number of reasons, the company could make a reduction to the total prize amount. I threw the card away and told Ma what the story was. She never would have fallen for something like that pre-dementia; in fact, she quite possibly would have written a letter to the company, criticizing them for their underhanded ways. She had written many such letters in her lifetime.

Shortly after that, I found out that she had recently signed up and paid for a sewer line insurance policy to cover her if her old sewer line had a problem. She was just being her lifelong proactive self. The way I found out is that the insurance company returned her check because she filled it out for the wrong amount. I threw all the paperwork away and called her and reminded her that she just had a portion of her sewer line replaced a couple years prior. Ironically, another portion of her sewer line caved in a year later. Unfortunately, because I'd disregarded and thrown away the sewer insurance paperwork, we now had to pay for the repairs out of ma's savings. Apparently, she was better at preparing for these types of events than I was, and I should have followed up with her original insurance plans.

THANKSGIVING 2013

Ma was at our house for Thanksgiving lunch. She became sad when it was time to take her home late in the afternoon. She asked me if I wanted to come up to her room for a bit and I said sure but not for too long because I was tired. She said that I could lay down there if I wanted. She was very lonely and just wanted company, so I stayed longer but eventually had to leave.

She asked me, "What exactly does this place (assisted living) do for me?"

"What are your long-term plans for me?"

"We're using up all my money (yet she had absolutely no idea what her financial situation was)."

She continually complained about being in assisted living, which I completely understood. She just could not accept that she was going to be there for the long term, not short, and it broke my heart. She refused to send any letters out using their outgoing mailbox. She refused to use the ALF as her return address. She refused to have me bring her sewing machine to her room (she had loved to sew for as long as I could remember). She refused to have her hair cut at the ALF salon. It was on-site and cheap, but she absolutely insisted that she had to go to her stylist over on the east side of town because, "they know how to do it."

On one hand, I was frequently frustrated, especially in the early weeks of the assisted living stage. On the other hand, I was proud of her for her stubbornness and refusal to lie down quietly. She fought it boy, she fought it with everything she had. She was going toe-to-toe with the heavyweight boxing champ of the world and, even though she took plenty of blows in the form of gradually losing her independent way of life and other indignities, she fought back bravely. It was admirable and, at the same time, very sad for me.

Later in the week, I stopped to visit with Ma after work. Our talk went fine for the first twenty minutes, right up until the time she said, "So, when are you getting me outta here?"

She argued with me for thirty minutes. "I lived in my own house for sixty years and I was just fine," she said.

"I don't have any money because this place is sucking me dry," she said.

"Just send me to Chicago," she said.

I said, "And where will you live when you're there, Ma?"

"Well, if you leave me here something's going to happen to me."

I said, "At least I've done everything I could to keep you safe."

"Then I'll just run away and you won't be able to find me."

I suggested that she bring plenty of warm clothes because we'd just had six days in a row with temperatures in the single digits. Then I explained that if I thought that she might do something like that, I'd have her put on lockdown. She didn't realize that the place she was in didn't have a lockdown service per se, although they did have a bracelet that would cause an alarm to go off if she tried to go out any of the main doors. I classified this as an acceptable white lie.

She told me that she wanted to straighten out the photo mess at her house, which consisted of thousands of photos she had taken over the years that were presently in complete disarray. It was a daunting project and she hadn't been able to get started on it for several years prior to assisted living. At one point, she wanted me to bring her several boxes of photos along with photo albums so that she could work on it. Eventually, she refused to do that and said it would have to wait until she lived back at her house.

She said she had just realized that the microwave in her room was hers from her house. She thought that it came with the room. She wanted me to take it out of there and put it back in her house, so it'd be there when she lived there again. She also wanted me to remove her plants and magazines for the same reason. She cried a little. She yelled a lot. She made many unhappy, disgruntled faces. She tried to make me out to be the bad guy (let's face it, I was). I told her that she couldn't scare, intimidate, or manipulate me, but boy-oh-boy did she try. She was still able to put up a mighty struggle while at the same time she was becoming more and more confused as her emotions ran wild and her mental capacity steadily decreased.

Overall, it wasn't a very pleasant visit for either of us. As I mentioned earlier, I was also confused with all that was going on and frequently felt as if I wasn't doing the right thing. She was struggling emotionally and cognitively, and I was trying to figure out the best way to deal with her problems as well as with my own perceived shortcomings of how I dealt with her. Dementia was having its way with both of us.

THIS IS MY MOM 12/12/2013

Ma complained frequently that she couldn't bake at the ALF and she missed it, so one day we provided the opportunity for her to do just that. We could have had her use our kitchen but felt that it'd be better if she could use the kitchen in her own house, where she was used to baking. We worked it out with one of our friends, a Certified Nursing Assistant (CNA), to pick up my mom from the ALF while Sandy and I were at work and take her there so she could have the home-kitchen advantage. For many years, she always made numerous types of Christmas goodies and sent them all over the country. Several years prior, she told me that she usually made as many as twenty-six different items. It was a tradition.

For the last year or two, she didn't consider the freshness of the ingredients that she used, and she also started to cut corners when it came time to include all the ingredients that the recipe called for. Some of the stuff tasted pretty nasty.

This was hard to swallow (pun intended) because she had been a wonderful baker in her prime. I especially liked the toffee, standard cutout cookies, and pfeffernuss cookies, which were one of her German mother's specialties. I always looked forward to these when I was a kid and into my adult years, right up to the time when she was not able to do it any longer. She'd bring the goodies over in a cookie tin and I'd demolish them.

For this event, Sandy pulled out two of Ma's recipe cards and laid out the ingredients so that Ma could make up the two batches. I talked to Ma the night before and told her that she'd have all the stuff she needed for making two types of cookies. When our friend brought her in the house, Ma went ballistic as to why there was only enough stuff present to make just two batches of cookies.

Our friend told her she would pick her up and have her back to the ALF by four. Instead, Ma called her at one p.m. and said she needed to go home because the baking session was over. When she got in the car she was, once again, livid about only having enough for two batches. As it turned out, she only made one batch. She just couldn't handle it and I assumed she was mad because she realized that she couldn't handle it. She generally complained about almost everything we tried to do for her, no matter what it was. This can start to wear on you after a while, but I kept trying anyway because I knew it wasn't her fault. It was Dementia's fault. The dementia which started out slowly, but gradually, then continually, increased.

It just kept coming.

It was relentlessly damaging and neither Ma, nor I, could keep up with it. More than once I'd decide to take a break for a few days, but then I'd ask myself, "How can I do that? This is my mom." Sure, she was in an assisted living facility where she was being looked after, but I'd learned early on that the unpredictable incompetence of the staff was one more issue I had to contend with. And I thought about all these issues, and more, every day. Every day. Every single day.

The reality is that there was NO break because even if I did skip visits every now and then, I couldn't shut it off in my mind. So, while Ma was unknowingly trying to keep her brain active and "normal," I was trying to shut mine off, at least for a little bit. In these regards, neither one of us was very successful.

The next day, I brought Ma to our house for a birthday party for two of our friends, both of whom she knew very well. On the way, we stopped outside the post office and mailed one hundred and thirty Christmas cards containing her Christmas letter. As I mentioned above, she refused to use the postal services at the ALF. And for that, kudos are in order because her canniness was uncanny. At some level, at least some of the time, she knew things weren't right with her thought processes and in these moments of partial clarity she'd come up with a new plan for distancing herself from any ties with the ALF. The post office idea certainly required a higher level of thought than I assumed she was capable of at the time. She was still slugging it out with the heavyweight champ and, occasionally, she'd land a solid blow.

Early in our visit, she asked me if she could have her credit card. I asked her why, and she said that in case she went somewhere and wanted to buy something she could pay for it and not have to carry cash. Remember, she wasn't driving at all. She did go on the ALF shuttle bus to Walmart once a week, but she didn't spend too much because she thought she was going broke. I made sure she always had forty or fifty dollars to spend. I told her I was leery of her buying something from a salesperson who might take advantage of her. I also told her I was worried about her losing the card, as she did with her keys, phone, and pepper spray, among other things.

She said, "Okay, honey."

Less than twenty minutes later, she came up to me at the party and said, "I'm really disoriented."

I said, "Let's you and I go sit down in the living room, because you're very comfortable there, and see how it goes."

We sat down on the very couch where she'd had her breakdown just two months before (it seemed like two years). She loved this couch because it was right in front of a large picture window that looked out over the big trees in my front yard with the sometimes-snow-covered Pikes Peak in the background. When she turned around, she was then able to see the fireplace, along with the piano and the dining area beyond that. It was her favorite place to sit when she was at my house.

I asked her if she wanted something to drink like coffee, tea, or wine. She took the wine and said that she was used to drinking that at night. As the night went on, her mental condition continued to deteriorate until she told me she was tired and, at seven thirty, she told me she was ready to go home. She had slouched shoulders and shuffled as she walked. Sometimes, she looked like her mother and other times I could imagine me looking like that when I became her age. It was always so heartbreaking for me to see her like this. I think she was just overwhelmed with the commotion, even though it was a small party. In the past, she always enjoyed these get-togethers very much. After she finished her glass of wine, she didn't want to say goodbye to anyone, so we quietly left the house and I took her home.

Two days later, Mom left the following message on my cell phone: "John, would you please get me outta here as soon as you can. I'm getting more depressed every day. Bye (She was crying a little)."

So was I.

WHERE'D THEY DIG YOU UP?

In mid-December, my brother Jim came from Illinois to visit and I had not mentioned to Ma that he was coming because I thought a surprise would be nice for her. So Jim, my oldest daughter and I went over to have supper with her. Kiddo went in first, followed by me, and I placed Jim kinda behind me so that Ma couldn't see him. After I hugged her, she then looked up and saw Jim. She paused for a minute and said, "Where'd they dig you up?"

She did recognize him, but I believe it was just barely. She didn't jump back and yell, "Oh my God!" or anything like that. She was quite subdued. We went to her room after dinner and were planning to bring her back to my house for the evening. Eventually I said, "Well Ma, are you ready to go?"

She said "Yeah, everybody grab a plant."

The rest of us all looked at each other, confused. She thought we were taking her over to her house to move back in, right then, and she wanted her plants to go with her. How she managed to come up with yet another escape plan was, and still is, unknown to me. It was cute, humorous, and tragic all at the same time. Once we cleared that up, I said again, "Well Ma, are you ready to go?"

"Where?"

"To my house," I said.

She said, "Forever?"

We finally made it to my house, and she wasn't there one hour and wanted us to take her home. She said she was uncomfortable. This was at my house, with my family and brother Jim there. As she requested, we took her back to the ALF.

All Downhill from Here

The next day, Jim took her over to her house so that she could make a couple batches of toffee. After the first batch she had to lie down because she was tired. Jim spent most of the afternoon with her and then brought her over to our house about four. I was half dozing on the recliner, watching a movie, and she came up behind me, tossed the Saturday newspaper on my lap, and in an angry tone said, "Here's your paper." (Six months prior, I had cancelled my newspaper subscription. After that, she liked to bring us her newspaper after she'd finished reading it.) This was not even close to normal behavior for her. Typically, she'd leave the paper on the kitchen counter, but on this day, she was acting like she was upset with me.

I was trying to finish the last fifteen minutes of a movie that I'd been watching for two hours when she sat down and brought a stack of all the Christmas cards she'd received at our house over the last several days. She felt like reciting every card to me while I was trying to watch the movie. She started reading to me, so I paused the movie and said, "Ma, I'm trying to finish this movie, but it can wait if you want to talk."

She threw up her hands in disgust and said nothing. I started the movie again and, two minutes later, she was waving a photo in front of my face and it showed several people of a large family that I'd never even heard of before. It was the family of a girlfriend of hers from elementary school. Once again, I explained I was trying to finish the movie but could stop if she wanted, and, once again, she threw up her hands in disgust.

Soon after that she said, "I think I'll just have Jim take me home."

I said, "Ma, I thought you wanted to come over for supper with us and you've been here less than thirty minutes and you want to leave, how come?"

She said, "It's five fifteen and I don't know where Sandy or the girls are and there's nobody to talk to."

"Ma, the clock you're looking at is wrong. Look at the clock on the wall behind you, it's only four thirty. You know we never eat this early."

Jim came over and said, "What's up, Ma?"

"It's five fifteen and I don't know where anybody is."

I said, "Ma, it's only four thirty. You're looking at the wrong clock."

Once again, she threw up her hands in disgust. At least she agreed to hold tight until we could get some chili in her. Taking her home, she saw Bonnie's restaurant and commented on the Christmas lights once again, as if it was the first time she'd seen them. This happened four nights in a row while Jim was in town and it must've been nice to see them as new every night. That'd have to be cool because I still enjoyed seeing them and I went by there all the time. I was glad she forgot that she was mad at me.

12/22/2013

Jim and I went to see Ma and she wanted to show us a recent treasure that she found on one of her recent walks. It was a black metal box she'd found in one of the stairwells in her building. It was about ten inches square by three inches high and on one end of it there was a hole. It looked like a mouse hole that you'd see in the wall of a Tom and Jerry cartoon. Closer inspection revealed that it was a humane mousetrap (it actually WAS a mouse hole). We told Ma about this and she was disappointed. She was planning to use the box for a container for her soon-to-be-baked Christmas cookies. We placed it back in the stairwell where she told us she'd found it.

In the mail she received a Christmas card from Bill and in the address, instead of saying "Room number 353," he wrote "Cell number 353." Ha!

At Ma's request, Jim looked for, and found, her magnifying glass in the bed blankets between the bed and the wall. She was amazed! Once again, she had blamed the cleaning man for taking it (as she had also done with her TV remote, phone, and pepper spray) and, once again, the primary suspect was acquitted. He was free to move about as he pleased. For now.

Eventually, it was time to take Jim to the airport. Ma walked us out to my truck, we hugged and said goodbye, and Jim and I sadly watched her walk back into the building. I had become somewhat used to our mom's behavior, as much as possible anyway. For Jim, it was shocking. He was visibly upset, looking out the window and not saying much as we drove to the airport.

CHRISTMAS DAY 2013

I told Ma the night before that I'd be over to get her in the morning at ten or so. I showed up at 10:10 and she practically jumped out of the chair in the lobby, where she had been waiting for me. She had already called the house looking for me, at 10:04. We got over to my house, where we had several presents for her from Bill and from us. I had bought her a small safe for keeping her valuables, which she could put in the lockable cabinet in her room. There was a fire in the fireplace and Christmas music was playing. She was generally happy.

After the presents, she handed me an old business card that my brother had made for her years earlier. It contained her name, address, email address, and phone number. She asked me if I could make several copies of it and I said, "Sure, what are you going to do with these, Ma?"

She said, "Oh, I want to give some of these to the people where I live now."

I said, "If the people where you live now want to get in contact with you, all they have to do is knock on your door."

She said, "No, this is for when I move out of there and go back to my house."

I admired her persistence and said, "Are you going to be moving out of there in the next coupla days?"

She said no.

I said, "Then I guess it's not a rush and I'll do it for you later, okay? Today's Christmas!"

And for the rest of the day that she was with us, say, six hours, she was pouting and in a sour mood. She just couldn't shake her bad feelings. It had to have been awful for her because not only did she like parties, but she especially liked the holidays. Before dementia, she would occasionally get in a down mood, like all of us, but she'd eventually shake it off and get on with things. That had changed. She was acting so very differently than we were used to and the "new normal" was becoming more and more frequent.

As planned, we went over to our friend's house, where more close friends joined us, all of whom she knew well. She barely said a word the whole time. This was so unlike her previous self that it caught all of us off guard. To reiterate, she had always loved these types of gatherings. She used to bring an entrée or two, along with the ever-present deserts that she loved to make. On this day, the beautiful holiday decorations glistened, with nice music in the background, great food, and lively conversation. It was Christmas Day, and she didn't enjoy one bit of it. Dementia was stealing her fun-loving spirit, along with her mental and physical abilities. Nevertheless, the rest of us had a ball. Sandy and I decided early on that, even though this was a rough disease for all concerned to deal with, we would do our best to keep our spirits up.

Sometimes it worked.

Afterwards, we took her home and as I walked her into the lobby of her place, I hugged her and said, "Ma, you have GOT to lighten up because you're making yourself miserable."

No response. She was so sad and upset that it was hard for her to talk. I had a lump in my throat as I kissed her on the head and said, "I love you, Ma."

As she slowly walked away, with the weight of her world on her shoulders, she didn't turn around to face me, but she did force out a weak, "I love you too, honey."

It was so hard to see her, once again, so sad and broken. Walking away and leaving her like this was never easy.

The next day, she called and left a message in high spirits, as if she hadn't had such a horrible time the day before. This is one of the few, if not the only, good things that occurred as the dementia continued – sure, she'd forget the good things that happened, but she'd also forget the bad things. She told me to come over the next morning as she had some things she wanted to discuss with me.

I called her the following day and she didn't even mention the high-energy message she'd left the day before. She did say that she sure hoped she'd get to see us one of these days. She said this frequently. I said, "Ma, we were just together for over six hours, two days ago."

She said, "I know, but I just get so lonely."

I said, "I know you do Ma, we're doing the best we can." I then explained that she was living at a place that housed over a hundred people in a similar situation to hers and that there must be at least a couple dozen people there that would have things in common with her. Nope. No dice. She continually dug in her heels and refused to do anything to help improve her situation.

2014 BEGINS

MY MOM, THE CRIMINAL

In early January, I went over to Ma's apartment to have lunch with her. It was a cold, gray, windy, slippery-roads kinda day. I had left her a message on her answering machine, but she didn't get it because she was busy dominating the bingo parlor, where she won quite often. I walked in just as she was exiting the bingo den filled with her latest victims. She looked pleased, in a sinister way, and asked me what I was doing there.

I had the Christmas safe and a few other things to bring up to her room and when we got there, I told her I was going to see how the safe fit in her cabinet so that I could get it mounted. She said, "We don't need that here, we can just bring it to my house." She held back a tear and then handed me the following letter that she had waiting for me:

John,

I've got to get out of here one way or another. I may end up in the hospital or jail, but I'll take that chance if need be.

I feel like I'm being punished. I feel like I've raised four great children with Dad's help. I love you all very much.

I'm grateful for all you've done for me.

I feel I can make it on my own in my house. I'm navigating quite well.

Maybe one of those medical alert buttons if you'll feel better.

I don't want to hurt you.

I love you and your family and want to see you.

Love, Mom

I said "End up in jail? Are you planning on busting up the bingo parlor?" She rarely saw the humor in my jokes anymore.

"Just tear it up," she said.

DEMENTIA'S IN CHARGE

We went down for lunch and she told me how her dining tablemate, Mary Lou, had just died the night before. She had recently taken a bad fall and hit her head, and then she fell again a few days later. Unfortunately, she passed away in the night. Mary Lou's husband, George, Ma's other tablemate, and his family were in a private room right next to where we were sitting, and Ma said quite loudly, "I never did like her very much anyway!"

Holy Cow! The poor woman wasn't even cold yet and my mom was flaming her in the dining room, less than fifty feet away from her grieving family members.

She said, "I just never liked the way she talked to George. She was just stupid."

I said, "Ma, she was sick. That's why she was here."

> **This is a prime example of "The dementia's in charge." My mom would never, ever, have acted like this before. Dementia doesn't just cause memory loss and cognitive decline. In this case it's easy to see that dementia was also slowly and steadily stealing her sense of kindness and compassion for others. It was a double whammy; her feelings of empathy were disappearing and at the same time she didn't have the cognitive ability to recognize it. She just kept drifting farther and farther away…….**

She didn't respond and wouldn't look me in the eye. She looked down at her trembling fingers as they fumbled with her napkin and moved her silverware around. She put quite a bit of time into finding something, or someone, to criticize.

We went for a little walk around the building and ran into George in his wheelchair. He was alone so it was a good time for me to hug him and offer my condolences. Poor man. I knew him fairly well and he was truly a kind and gentle person. He seemed to be taking it okay, but you never know what's going on inside. Ma didn't say anything to him as she walked me out to my car and pleaded with me to find a way to get her out of there while conversely, I was glad that she was in there and relatively safe.

A few days later, my family and I had supper with her at the ALF. She told me that Aunt Mary was going to send her a copy of the family tree and that she wanted it because she wanted to make some changes to it. That sounded good to me, although I doubted if she'd even be able to understand it, much less modify it. She said that she asked Aunt Mary to mail it to her house. I said, "Why didn't you have her send it here, to assisted living?" She said because she was hoping she wasn't going to be a resident for that long.

And then she said that she hated her new server in the dining room. She also hated the hobbled over old man who always had drool and stuff coming out of his mouth. She said she went for a walk behind the apartment buildings again. I told her that I'd asked her before not to walk behind the apartments but to stay out in plain sight. She said I'd never told her that before. "Alright, Ma," I said.

Later that week I went and met her for breakfast. She was very jumpy and ordered her food before anyone else at the table. Then she tried to order mine, too. The fact that she didn't know what I wanted made it difficult. I met her new tablemate, Margie, and I instantly liked her. She was quite old and kinda hunched over, but her mind was reasonably present. I could tell that she was intelligent, and she was still well-spoken.

George was there in his wheelchair and was his usual pleasant self. I told Ma that an old friend of hers had sent a letter to my house. I asked her if she remembered Priscilla and she looked amazed that she knew anyone by that name. I explained that Priscilla once lived across the street from us when I was seven years old, and she had a little girl the same age as me. The little girl and I planned on getting married. That's about all I could remember.

In her purse-of-things, she kept at least one copy of her enormous address list and she frantically searched for this alleged friend of hers named Priscilla. She'd scan down one page, then on to the next one, then back and forth through the whole thing. While she was on the hunt, I was talking to George and my new friend, Margie. Eventually, I could see Ma out of the corner of my eye, and she was holding her finger on the address list. She then filled me in on her new, old friend Priscilla and as she was doing so, she started to remember things about her and the things that they used to do together. She remembered that they had played cards all the time and that Priscilla had kids about the same age as my siblings and me.

Later in the breakfast, she said that she had a DVD she wanted me to watch. It was a travel film about Canada, and she said it was beautiful. She mentioned that she hoped Bill would take her to Canada some time and if he didn't, by God, she'd go by herself. I asked her how she'd get there, and she said, in a very matter-of-fact voice, "I'll drive."

"Sounds good, Ma."

After breakfast, we went up to her room and she told me about how much she hated this one woman in the dining room. I said, "Why do you hate her, Ma?"

"Because she's a bitch!" she said, as if everybody already knew that.

"Have you ever talked to her?"

"No."

"Then how do you know she's a bitch?"

"I just know," she said.

Once again, what I wanted to know was, what was happening to my mom? She was continually changing, literally, right before my eyes. She never would have made such a rude comment about this woman and even if she had felt that way, she wouldn't have said it in the condescending manner that she just used. I was shocked, but she acted as if this was just normal conversation. The anger and frustration she carried around, because of her new unwanted lifestyle, along with the unrelenting advance of dementia, was showing itself more frequently. And it was becoming harder to have anything resembling a normal conversation with her. She was never one to cuss very often but now, as the dementia worsened, she'd sometimes blurt out some real cuss-bombs.

I thought I'd change the subject, so I told her that I liked her new tablemate, Margie. It turned out that she hated Margie too. I asked her why and she said, "Because she's always staring at me."

She had mentioned this to me before. I said, "Ma, I watched Margie several times today and sometimes she looked at her food, sometimes at George or me, sometimes off in space. However, I never saw her look at you, much less stare. Maybe she's hard of hearing and, when she thinks you're about to say something, she stares so that she can read your lips. Or something like that."

"Well, I just don't like her."

Then she brought up the driving issue again and asked if she could just take a test to prove that she could drive to Canada. I told her there was no test that she could take that would cause me to let her drive again. Naturally, she wanted to know why, and I told her because she became confused easily and I wasn't sure that she knew where she was in her own town anymore, much less in another country.

Towards the end of my stay, we were in her room and she said, "I wish you weren't so hard on me."

Huh? What? I was stunned.

"Ma, how can you say that I'm hard on you? If I were hard on you, I'd take you to some nasty dump of a nursing home and drop you off. We'd never talk to you or come see you. I'd spend all your money and sell your house and you'd never see me again. I wouldn't take care of your bills or your taxes or your medical stuff, or anything else. That's not a very nice thing to say, Ma." And right after I said it, I felt like a major jerk, once again. It was the exact opposite of how I should have responded to her. As she was tumbling down the dementia staircase, I was trying to adapt, although I wasn't always making these changes to my behavior as quickly as I would have liked.

She was acting as if she were in Stalag 17 or a Siberian prison camp or the like (which, in her mind, she was) in yet another vain effort at coming up with valid reasons as to why she should be able to go home. At least that's what I think she was trying to do. At times, I found myself questioning my own sanity and wondering if dementia was contagious. She said, "You can leave now if you want. I know you have lots of stuff to do."

She was giving me the boot, which also was completely out of character for her up until dementia arrived. I knew it wasn't her talking, but it still hurt. We talked for a few more minutes and then I told her that I needed to go home and get busy. She said, "Wait. I have a bag that you might be able to use."

This was such a funny and cute thing for her to do, always giving my brothers and me various containers. I remember her saying several times over the previous forty years that, "Your dad always told me to save him any containers I ended up with." It didn't matter if it was a cookie tin, plastic box, cloth bag, or whatever. Ma saved them all. Dad would use them to store pipe fittings, sheet metal screws, and other miscellaneous pieces of hardware and fishing supplies.

She then brought out this big, clear plastic bag that she had stashed in her closet and, inside of it, there was a black canvas bag, approx. 36" X 18" X 6" high. There was writing on it that spelled Fortex. I asked her where she got it, but she didn't remember. I looked inside and there was a set of instructions for a Fortex Evacuation Chair of some sort. I wondered if this came from the stairwell. We went to the stairwell and right at the top of the landing was this big, black, folded up, plastic chair-looking-thing mounted to the wall. It was for the emergency evacuation of residents that weren't able to walk. And printed on the side of it, in big, white letters, was the word "Fortex." We left the bag right underneath it and went down the stairs. On the way down, we passed the mousetrap that was almost a cookie container.

I was beginning to sense a pattern.

ONE EXTRA POUND

Later in the week, Ma had a quarterly checkup with her primary care doctor. First, I had breakfast with her at the ALF and noticed that she had on these lightweight, flat, hard-soled black shoes with no tread. I told her she should wear her hiking boots, because it was very cold (twelve below), and there was ice and packed snow on the ground. We went to her room and she laced up the hiking boots. As we walked out the door, I saw that she was carrying her slippery black shoes. "What are you bringing those for, Ma?"

"Because I'll change into these before I go into the doctor's office and then I won't weigh as much."

And she really meant it. She had always been somewhat obsessed with keeping her weight down, but now she was seventy-eight years old, suffering from dementia, and still concerned about weighing what, one extra pound? And darned if she didn't remember to pull the ol' shoe switcheroo as we got closer to the doctor's office. It seemed odd to me that she remembered these kinds of things, yet she couldn't remember what to do in an airport.

For the doctor appointment, she was dressed very nicely, which was her style. She could, and did, get grubby when she was working in her yard, which she loved to do, but she was generally in a nice stylish outfit. Green and turquoise were her favorite colors, as well as shades near teal and chartreuse. As I mentioned earlier, earrings were generally part of the ensemble as well. I have very little fashion sense, and I'm certainly not qualified to comment on women's fashion in any way, but I know what looks nice. And my mom usually looked nice.

We stopped at her house on the way to the doctor because she wanted to drop some items off from her apartment that she "didn't need anymore." Books and things. She talked about it several times at breakfast, you know, how she "just wanted to go home." When we got to her house, she just threw the bag of books on the floor and said, "I'll straighten this up once I get back home."

After fifteen minutes of sitting on the couch and looking out the window she said, "I'm ready anytime, honey."

"Ma, we just got here, and you want to leave right away?"

Then she went on about just how much she needed to "straighten up" her house when she was living there again. As we were getting ready to go out the front door, she turned toward the kitchen and said, "Bye house." It wasn't an unusual thing to say in her position, but what was unusual was how she said it. You see, it was her pronunciation, not the words themselves. She sounded like a three-year-old that had recently learned how to pronounce "house." This is not a criticism of her in any way. It's what she sounded like. A child. In fact, in many of her actions she was beginning to act like a child. This, also, is not a criticism, just an observation. As we were driving away, she said it again.

"Bye house."

Ma loved her house in Colorado Springs, on the southwest corner of Essex and Alpine. I had arranged the purchase for her (she wired the funds) in 2000 while she was still living in Oak Lawn, IL. As far back as I could remember, she said that she wanted a red brick house, so I found one that met my criteria for condition, safety, and location. It was a ranch-style house, with a basement, built in 1961. She insisted on a place with a basement because she'd always had a basement, and that was that.

Oak Lawn, IL was the site of a deadly F4 tornado on April 21, 1967. We didn't move there until November 1967, but there were still signs of the tornado that I can remember quite well, even though I was only eight years old at the time. There were several trees on the edge of our yard and a clothesline pole had been pulled out of the ground and then hurled right through the trunk of one of the trees, like a harpoon. The cement that had held the pole in place when it was in the ground was still attached to the base of the pole and was there when I joined the Army and left home in 1977.

I can remember the sound of tornado sirens going off several times when I was young. And I vividly recall Mom and Dad carrying us four little kids down to the basement in the middle of the night, more than once. The wind was howling, and the tornado siren was blaring away, scaring me to death. Angry winds just on the other side of the wall. Pitch black except for the flashlights and the lightning flashes. I also remember several tornadoes during the day.

I remember the green sky.

2014 Begins

Maybe that's why she wanted a basement, even though tornadoes are very rare in Colorado Springs.

The main level of my mom's house had hardwood floors in every room, except for the kitchen and bathroom. The kitchen and bathroom were a bit dated, so I remodeled them within three years after she moved in. The house was in a wonderful central location, in a quiet neighborhood where big maple trees and colorful crab apple trees were the norm. She loved plants and flowers and had them throughout the house, along with many of her framed photographs. There was a large screened-in porch off the dining room and in the summer, she'd move many plants out to the porch. There was a huge picture window in the living room where she loved to sit and look outside. In the wintertime, when the leaves had fallen, Pikes Peak was visible to the west. The three gigantic maple trees in the back yard produced a large amount of leaves and in the fall, when my kids were little tykes, I'd rake together a huge pile of fallen leaves for them to dive into. Sometimes Susan across the back, and her young son Michael, would come over and join the fun. There was an old red and white metal shed in the corner of the yard that was kinda falling apart and the doors were hard to slide open. The only concern I had when selecting this house was that the back yard had quite a slope to it. When Ma first moved in, she insisted on cutting the grass and I was concerned about her pushing the lawn mower on the slope. It didn't bother her though, and she soldiered on as she was prone to do. She always wanted to live out West, and eventually she was able to do it. In her red brick house on Essex Lane.

On our way to the doctor's office, I was sure that she would bring up the subject of driving. She used to say how much she loved to "Go, go, go." Therefore, now that she couldn't drive anymore, it was very hard for her to accept the fact that she had to "Stop, stop, stop." She didn't mention it though, and I sure wasn't going to bring it up.

We walked into the examination room at the doctor's office and she whipped out her usual list of questions. The apple doesn't fall far from the tree because I also do this when I go to the doctor. The doctor was generally pleased with her status, although the blood pressure was still a bit high. I didn't understand this. When she first went into assisted living, the medicine techs there said that her doctor had sent orders to lower the strength of her blood pressure medication. As a result of the medication change, her blood pressure had been quite high ever since. I asked him if we could ever expect her blood pressure to be great at 110/70 or 120/80 or some such, and he said, "Sure."

Huh?

Anyway, he increased the dosage of one of her blood pressure medications and I told him we'd give it a month or so and call him if it was above 130/80. Then she asked him if her memory would ever get better and he thought about it and said, "You seem to be doing well in assisted living. You've gained ten pounds because you're eating regularly and you're staying busy with many different activities. So, once we get your blood pressure dialed in I think, sure, your memory could get better."

Now, I admit that I hadn't studied or investigated dementia. Nevertheless, I was quite sure that the disease did not get better. Therefore, I assumed he told her that because either, One: Why not give her something to hope for and, Two: She's going to forget that he said it, anyway. Either way, I saw this as "no harm done." Then she asked him when she'd be able to drive again. Once again, he thought on the question for a minute before responding, "Well, for starters you'd have to take a driver's test."

This perked her up briefly until John the Devil interjected with "Dr. John says that, no matter how you do on any driver's test, I just can't let you drive again, Ma."

She looked at me with teary eyes and pleaded, "But why?"

2014 Begins

After I recovered from the "punched in the solar plexus" feeling, I explained how we'd talked about this dozens of times and that she would not be driving again. She was then mad at me for at least a minute before she forgot about it and then moved on to her next item of concern and said, "Doc, when will I be able to live in my house again?"

Now, with this one, he took an extra-long time before answering. Finally, he came up with, "Assisted living seems to agree with you, and you seem to be thriving there. You need to look at this as a long-term situation."

Not exactly what she wanted to hear, I assure you. She was trying hard to get him to take her side and give her the green light. That didn't happen, and he ended up taking my side, which was not in her plan book. My goal above anything else was to keep her as safe as possible, but she didn't look at it that way. The doc then stated that he thought she was doing fine, and that he'd make the necessary changes to her blood pressure medicine. Then he asked her, "So Nancy, how's your memory?"

She said, "Good. It's generally good."

Huh? Nobody was looking at me, but I did roll my eyes. Her memory is generally good? Holy cow. Her memory had degraded to the point that she didn't know that her memory was bad. I had brought a magazine into the exam room with me and it was in my lap. I saw another one on a counter top next to the doctor, so I just stood up and said, "Excuse me, Ma, I need to put this magazine over here before I forget."

I put the magazine away and turned to the doc and whispered, "Her memory is terrible," and sat back down. I didn't want to mention it in front of Ma and hurt her feelings, but I felt that the doctor needed to hear the real story.

He responded to her statement and told her, "Good. Good. Glad to hear it."

Then he asked her how her mood was. Was she happy, sad, or maybe lonely sometimes? She said, "Good. Yep. Pretty good."

Double eye roll. Holy cow. It blew me away just how removed from reality she really was. Once again, he said, "Good. Good. Glad to hear it. Let's say we see you again in about three months, okay?"

"Okay."

I asked her if she could go out to the waiting room so that I could talk to the doctor alone for a few minutes, which she did. When we were alone, I told him about her terrible memory and how it was progressively getting worse. He said he understood and commented that this was the general course of dementia. There really wasn't a whole lot that we could do. Then I told him about her generally horrible mood. She was kinda mean and nasty when speaking to other residents. She was very short with them. She was down in the dumps more often than not, yet sometimes manic. Sometimes lucid and usually anxious. However, the depression was the biggest problem, because she tended to get so low. He said, "Maybe it's time we get her on an antidepressant."

That sounded good to me and then I mentioned that she had been to a therapist recently and that I had arranged this in the first place with the sole intent of maybe getting her on an antidepressant. I asked him if he thought going to the therapist again would do her any good. Me, I didn't think she'd tell the therapist the truth about her mental issues anyway. He said, "Not only that, but with her dementia, she wouldn't remember anything the therapist told her to work on."

Touché.

I then went on about how, when this all started and she was so down, that I'd rather have her drugged up and somewhat happy then drug free and miserable. I qualified my "drugged up" comment with the fact that I was using the term as a figure of speech and that I didn't intend for it to be clinically accurate. He understood and said that she wouldn't appear "drugged up" per se, but that she would be happier and calmer, which sounded good to me. I said that I'd want to start her out on a small dose and see how things went and he agreed.

In early February, I took the kids and one of their friends to have dinner with Ma at the ALF and she said, "When you get a chance, can you get a gallon of wine and put it in my fridge?"

"Ma, a bottle that big won't fit in your fridge here."

She yelled, "Yes it will! I've done it lots of times!!!"

"What fridge are you talking about, Ma?"

"The one in my house."

I said, "Ma, you heard the doctor the other day. Assisted living is a long-term situation. This is your house for right now, remember?"

She was mad at me again for a minute or two. As I mentioned previously, in some cases it was good that her memory wasn't great because she'd forget some, or all, of the things I said that she disagreed with. I continually had to contend with how fast she was failing, how I had a hard time accepting it, and how I'd sometimes incorrectly deal with her rapidly changing situation. I don't think that I was intentionally in denial, but a part of me still felt that this wasn't real. But at the same exact time I knew that she'd never be back, regardless of what I thought or did. We both continued to struggle with the never-ending changes that occurred.

After I returned home, I was busy with gathering the pertinent income tax forms and documents as I prepared for an appointment with my CPA for the annual bloodletting. In conjunction with this task over the years, I also chose this as the time to evaluate our overall financial picture. At this point, I had been taking care of my mom's finances for some time as well, so I also decided to evaluate her overall financial picture at the same time. I was concerned that her finances had taken quite a hit due to a few big-ticket expenses, in addition to her monthly assisted-living-costs. For the record, I'm a very conservative investor and have steered clear of the stock market for several years. I'm very risk-averse. On the other hand, my mom had various investments including mutual funds and individual stocks, that I feared had suffered due to the various market downturns that occurred since I'd last reviewed her overall portfolio.

Imagine my surprise when I discovered that her investments related to the stock market had appreciated substantially! Her buy-and-hold strategy, which happened without any formal planning on her part, had turned out just great. She was not necessarily a savvy investor, but she owned stocks that she had inherited from her mother, as well as a few IRA mutual funds that she had acquired from various employers over the years. In short, my seventy-eight-year-old mother with dementia, and no knowledge of stock market tactics, was a better investor than me.

The following week I had dinner with my daughter and Mom at the ALF. Ma said, "Bill sure wants to see those great grandkids (her oldest granddaughter had just given birth to identical twin girls). He said he'd drive here from California and then we'll go to Illinois and pick up Mary Ann (my sister). Then, we'll go down to Austin and see the babies. Then, we'll go back to Illinois and bring Mary Ann home. Then, we'll come back to Colorado and then he'll go back to California."

"Holy cow, Ma. You're talking 6-7000 miles here, are you sure Bill's on-board with this? Does he have a vehicle that Mary Ann will be able to get in and out of, maybe with a wheelchair?"

She then whispered to me, discretely, so that the secret didn't leak out, "He's got a new car. It's a Cadillac."

'nuff said.

I said, "Well, that amount of mileage is something like one quarter the circumference of the earth, are you sure Bill's up for it?"

"Well, he said he was."

She also asked me when she'd be able to live in her house again. I reminded her that her doctor said that she needed to look at assisted living as a long-term situation, but she had no recollection of him saying that. I wasn't sure if she was starting to make peace with these kinds of things, or what. Maybe she just forgot about them shortly after they were discussed? I suspected the latter, because making peace with something that she strongly opposed was, typically, not in her repertoire.

2/16/2014

I talked to Bill and asked him about his upcoming trip going one quarter of the way around the earth and he laughed and said that he had been joking with her when he said that. As it turned out, he was planning on taking the train to Colorado and then using either my mom's car or my truck, which he'd then take down to Austin. His and Ma's two versions of the plans for the trip jived except for the total length of the trip, the mode of transportation to/from Colorado, the vehicle they'd drive from Colorado and the number of passengers on board. This type of confusion would never have occurred before my mom's dementia because she always had her plans laid out very precisely. Not anymore.

The next day I stopped to see Ma after work, and she was complaining about assisted living again. I asked her how her lunch went the day before, with her nephew Tim and his wife Anne, from Boulder, CO (100 miles north of Colorado Springs). She said it was good, but right after that she told me she had to call Aunt Mary to find out whose son Tim was. I couldn't find a way to joke with her about this.

Later in the week, I went to dinner with the kids at the ALF. We were fifteen minutes late and Ma was calling on the phone as we walked in the front door, even though I'd told her we might be late. We went in the private dining room, which adjoined the main dining area, and she was frantic because we didn't have any menus. She said that she hoped to be out of there by St. Patrick's Day (approximately one month away). She couldn't participate in our conversations that evening at all and merely waited for a break in the action before she'd jump in with whatever was in her mind from the last time she spoke during the previous break in the action. She could hold on to that one thought, but that was about it. I tried to talk to her several times, about things that she used to be interested in, to no avail. We all went up to her room afterwards and she told me that she had to call a woman who'd sent her a letter, but she couldn't remember who it was. Then she asked me, "Did I ever work in San Francisco?"

I said, "Yeah, sure Ma, you worked there for many years when you volunteered for the park service, remember?" I continued, "You were right by the Golden Gate Bridge, Alcatraz, and Muir Woods. You worked for Teri and had a room of your own in a large house in the forest."

"Oh yeah, that's right," she said. This perked her up a bit and she flashed a brief smile as she recalled the good times that she had in northern California.

At times, I would treat these memory lapses as nothing out of the ordinary, even though they were. Logically, I was aware that the mom I'd known my whole life was fading away before my eyes, but sometimes I'd still pretend that this wasn't the case. At the same time, she would sometimes act with a degree of coherence that indicated that maybe she was getting better, even though she wasn't. I was holding on to a memory that was disappearing right in front of me.

WHAT IF I WIN A MILLION DOLLARS?

A few days after that, I had breakfast with Ma at the ALF. Afterwards, we went up to her room and visited for a while. Almost every time I was there, she told me that she wanted me to take something from her room and bring it over to her house. This time it was a pair of shoes that she asked me to remove. "What for, Ma?" I asked.

"It's because I want to make it easier on you when the time comes to move me out of here."

Was she being sarcastic? Was she being altruistic? Was she trying to deceive me? With her limited mental powers, I can't accurately say what caused her to think that way. If she was trying to deceive me, you had to admire it. Out of curiosity, I asked her when she thought she'd be living in her house again, but she didn't respond because she was on to the next matter of importance. She was angrily pulling out her new phone book and then she put on her mean face. She was mad, she was on a mission, and it was game-on.

"I can't believe that the new phone book doesn't have my address listed as 2224 Essex Ln. I looked it up yesterday and they listed my address as the address for this place." She was referring to the address at the assisted living facility.

"Seems kinda like a normal thing to do, Ma. This is where your phone is, and this is where they send the bill. You don't have to show it to me though, I believe you."

She kept trying to find her name in the phone book, so she could show it to me. "Well I don't like it and I want you to get it changed."

The name search continued. "I want you to call them up and make sure it never happens again."

"Sounds good, Ma. I'll do that next year because the phone book only comes out once a year.

"There it is!" She jumped up with her finger marking the spot and positioned it in front my face, "See. See."

"You got it, Ma. But I'm not sure why this bothers you so much?"

"Because what if I move back home and then I win a million dollars? If they look me up in the phone book, they'll send it to this place and I won't get it."

"But Ma, if that happens I'm sure the money people will be very diligent and sure about where they're sending your million dollars. Plus, if it comes here and you're living at your house, the post office will forward it to you." I don't know if that satisfied her or not, but she dropped the subject.

A few weeks earlier, she received a gift from her friend, George. It was a wonderful hand-made clock. Prior to becoming a resident at the ALF, he had been an avid woodworker. Shaped like a large arrowhead, the whole piece had a Native American theme, with small drawings of feathers and an adobe house in the background, on top of a base coat of glossy black paint. Beautiful. Ma told me to, "Get it out of here."

Apparently, the assisted living theft cartel was up to its old tricks again and she wasn't interested in becoming just another statistic. I then brought it to my house with the intention of eventually bringing it over to her house, for safekeeping. It was in a plastic grocery store bag, along with 60-70 Christmas cards that she'd received (via my mailbox) and wanted to save. She had taken the cards out of their envelopes and put the envelopes in the bag as well. I took them home and set them on top of the hutch right next to where she sat at our supper table. It's where I put things that needed to go to the ALF, or to take to her house when I went there to water the plants and keep an eye on the place. It was the grandma staging area

SPRING 2014

In early March, Sandy brought Ma to our house for supper (I was at work). When Ma sat down at the supper table, she noticed that there were items in her staging area. She opened the bag and said, "What a nice clock. I guess John wants me to take it back to my room. Oh look, there're Christmas cards in here, too."

She took the cards out of the bag, looked at several of them, and said, "I wonder why he didn't leave them in the envelopes, now I'm not going to know who they're from." She then took the clock and Christmas cards with her, back to her apartment, completing the round trip. I pondered on it for quite a while and realized that I was beginning to adjust to this type of behavior, which was quite a contrast when compared to the extremely organized woman I'd known all my life.

A couple weeks later, I was visiting with her one evening and she said that her blood pressure was still nice and low and that we should make copies of her readings for the doctor. I asked to look at the numbers and saw that they certainly were nice and low. I had told her doctor that I'd call his office only if her numbers were consistently above 130/80, and they weren't, so there was no reason to call him. She still wanted to make copies of the numbers to bring with us on our next visit with him. I told her that'd be fine, but I did ask her why.

"Because then he'll see that my blood pressure is good enough and then I can go back home."

Then she said that she hadn't gone to Walmart again, even though the shuttle bus went over there every Tuesday. She used to go every week but had skipped the last three. I asked her why and she said she just didn't feel like it, but she would like to go if Sandy or I would take her. I said, "Well, I don't go there very often, Ma, but I'll sure take you if you want to go. Why don't you try the bus next week and see how it goes?" I thought that the outings on the bus would be good for her.

She responded quickly with "Whatever," as she turned her head away and dropped the subject. I think she was starting to have a hard time deciding what to do or where to go, when she was in the store. In her pre-dementia state, she frequently said that she "hated shopping," but that sure didn't stop her from going! She didn't spend much time at the higher-end stores, but she loved going to second-hand stores such as Goodwill and the like. She liked to "rummage around," especially when it was senior discount day. Lately, even that was becoming too difficult for her to manage.

I was visiting with her a few days later and she did her usual rundown of the day's activities. Exercise, bingo, live music. She then mentioned the six people that she talked with on the phone in the past twenty-four hours, but she was still bored and there wasn't anything new. "Just trying to stay busy," she said.

Then she added, "Oh yeah, I haven't called Gramma yet."

I said, "Gramma who?"

"Gramma Shanahan." (She was talking about her mother). She said this as if the fact that she was talking about her mother should have been common knowledge. It seemed as if she had to exercise quite a bit of restraint to keep from saying "duh," as she explained it to me.

I said, "Ma, Gramma Shanahan's been gone for twenty-five years, how could you call her?"

She paused for just a second and looked so sad as her shoulders slumped. Then she looked me right in the eye and came back with, "Well, you know I don't think so straight anymore."

"That's okay, Ma. You were probably just thinking about her today or maybe you were talking to someone about her or something like that."

"Whatever."

Her sister and brother-in-law were coming from Illinois in a couple weeks and none of us were sure how she would handle it. It wasn't clear whether she was planning on leaving assisted living temporarily and staying at her house with them, or what. I asked, "So, what are you planning on doing when Aunt Mary and Uncle Jim are here?"

This threw her for a loop, and then she started moving her lips, but no sounds were coming out. She started to get anxious and nervous and didn't know what to say. She was rubbing her hands together and it was clear that she was quite confused. I said, "Take your time Ma, there's no rush."

Finally, she said, "Oh, we can go shopping and stuff like that. And make sure they have a key for my house." It was very important for her to make sure that Aunt Mary and Uncle Jim had a key for her house. I know that it was important because she mentioned it to me 673 times!

Then she told me about her new dining mate, Cheryl, who lived in Colorado Springs and was going to be leaving soon. I said "Leaving? Where's she going?"

Ma threw her arms up and said, matter-of-factly, "Goin' home." She acted as if everyone was going home but her, which was easy to understand given her situation.

As I mentioned above, for many years she told anyone who'd listen just how much she hated shopping. She absolutely hated it. Then, when people would come to visit, she'd take them shopping whether they wanted to go or not. I was beginning to piece together the contradiction that existed between how she thought of herself, or how she wanted others to perceive her, and how she really was. I'm no student of psychology, but it seems likely to me that we all do this to some degree or other. But when you have dementia, you're apparently no longer able to disguise it.

In late March, I went to visit Ma and needed to perform changes of address on her recurring bills so that the statements would come to my house, instead of hers. During the phone calls with the various companies, it was sometimes necessary for me to hand the phone to Ma, so that she could give her permission for the person to talk to me concerning her account. When I first got there, she was waiting for me in the lobby and as soon as I saw her I noticed the mentally ill look in her sunken eyes, or maybe it was behind her sunken eyes. Her skin was pale, and she was shaking. She was clearly depressed and upset. When we got up to her room, she whipped out the recent blood pressure numbers and, once again, brought up about how she wanted to show these to the doctor so that she could leave the ALF. She said, "Please get me out of here, for my sanity."

"What would you do if you were at your house, Ma?"

"Oh, I'd sew. And bake."

"How about if I bring your sewing machine here," I suggested.

She yelled, "No! I won't sew when I'm here!"

I switched subjects and asked her if she remembered what year it was when her mother had passed away. I was trying to determine when she had inherited shares of stock from her mom because I needed the information for preparing her income tax returns. She couldn't remember when her mom had passed away, so I told her that was fine and that I'd check with Aunt Mary. This helped her shift gears to the manic side and resulted in her retrieving her lengthy list of birthdays and anniversaries. Although she couldn't find what I was looking for, this did give rise to a long discussion concerning many, many birthdays.

She was like a kid in a candy store! "Oh look, my dad would have been one hundred and twelve on his next birthday. And tomorrow is so-and-so's birthday, ha ha!"

I didn't know many of the people that she was talking about, but this didn't matter because she wasn't talking to me anyway. I just happened to be in the room and I'm the one who provided the spark to get her goin'. It was great to see her in such a happy mood and I kept quiet as she enjoyed herself.

I still had one company to call to set up the change of address. She then told me that she wanted to get a haircut and she thought it was $13.50. She was talking about getting a haircut on-site and not at the special salon across town! It dawned on me that ever since she'd quit going to Walmart, she hadn't asked for any money. No big deal, it was her money after all. It was just an observation. Then she said, "Well, you can come to lunch with me now or we can go out."

I explained that I'd just had a molar pulled and didn't have much of an appetite but that I'd walk down and sit with her during lunch as soon as I made the last phone call. And just like that, she was back in depressed mode. She lowered her head and said, "Well if we're gonna go, we should go."

I reiterated that I needed to make just one more call.

"It's 11:30," she said. It wasn't a statement, it was a command. Mealtime was very much a lockstep routine for her, as were many other structured events that the ALF wisely provided. Even though she "wasn't a big eater, and never had been," (this was a comment she made frequently for as long as I could remember) she was very concerned about getting to the dining room at a specific time and not eating much.

I said, "Let me just make this last call and then we'll roll."

She put away the list and the darkness continued to descend on her like a cold blanket. I could see her mood spiraling down while I talked on the phone. After finishing the phone call, I picked up the newspapers waiting for me by the door and we left. I gave her a hug and she kissed me on the cheek and, through her tears said, "Thanks for all you do for me, honey."

After she'd eaten her lunch, I held back my own tears and took another sad walk to the parking lot.

4/6/2014

My mom's sister and brother-in-law arrived from Illinois. I was at work when they stopped by my house and picked up a key for, and directions to, Ma's house. The next day we all had lunch together at my house, along with my cousin Tim and his wife Anne. Ma was acting very distant to everybody and, even though everyone else around the table was laughing and kidding around, she went over to the couch and sat there by herself. Before dementia, she would have been joking along with everyone else because this was a crowd she knew well. Tim went and talked with her on the couch, but she never joined the group. She just wasn't comfortable with it. In fact, she was ready to leave right after we ate. "We can go anytime, honey," she said.

I gave her a hug and said, "Ma, do you know what everyone in this room has in common?"

She said no.

I said, "They all love you very much."

And boy did that get a big smile out of her! And then she reiterated, "We can go anytime, honey."

We stayed at my house for a couple hours longer, with me hoping that some of her old self would surface. Nope. She stayed in her down mode and I eventually took her back to the ALF late in the afternoon.

The next day, she did manage to talk Uncle Jim into taking the microwave out of her assisted living room and bringing it back to her house. Aunt Mary told me that they went back to Ma's apartment later in the day and Ma was complaining that she didn't have any way to make hot water so that she could have a cup of tea in her room.

On Tuesday, Aunt Mary and Uncle Jim went over to Ma's apartment to take her to lunch before they went back to Chicago. Ma decided it'd be best if they just headed for home without taking her to lunch because she was concerned about the weather, so Aunt Mary and Uncle Jim visited with Ma while she ate her lunch and then they headed for home. I suspected that she might have been so uncomfortable around people, just about any people, because she thought everyone expected her to act as she always had. Or something like that.

The following week I went to see Ma after work on Tuesday, as usual. She told me that her friend George's sister was now a resident at the assisted living facility. I asked her if that meant that there'd be a new dinner friend at their table to join Margie, George, and her. She said, "No. Her husband is in here too and I don't think he and George get along. Anyway, there's only one empty seat and, well, maybe after I leave they can both sit at the table together."

We then made small talk for a few minutes when, unexpectedly, she said, "George's sister is quite ugly."

Without missing a beat, she then said, "Margie's planning on staying here for the rest of her life."

Then she said, "I think George is going to go home any time now."

"Ma, George is well into his eighties. I'm guessing he doesn't drive. His wife recently passed away and he's in a wheelchair. He's probably here for the long haul, right?"

But mentally, she had already left the table. She was starting to spend more time staring off into space, at nothing in particular. She wouldn't say a word and sat like that for several minutes at a time. Sometimes a noise would catch her attention, and her head would jerk towards the sound. Sometimes she closed her eyes.

In early April, I was having breakfast with her and she looked mentally ill again. Bad. It was as if she had partially deflated. She hunched over slightly, she was shaking, and her sunken eyes looked almost black. She had always had such sparkling blue eyes but now the blueness was fading away. Regardless of that, she still managed to hurry us to her table, where we had places to sit because Cheryl's newly vacated seat was empty and George's ugly sister hadn't had a chance to sit down yet. She was so anxious that **I** had trouble sitting still.

I carried on with George and Margie for a few minutes. When I talked to Ma she was fine, but, once again, she wasn't able to contribute to any of the conversation that was going on around the table. If I asked her opinion on something that I was talking to one of the others about, she would act annoyed and give a very short answer. She was clearly unhappy, alternately manic and depressed and not thrilled with the menu. Right after breakfast we went up to her room. I had some income tax forms for her to sign and we got that done right away. Then she brought up the subject of Bill coming out and then taking her to Austin to see the great-grandbabies.

She said, "Bill's coming in late April or early May and we need to get three weeks of my medication to take with us."

Now, for the last year or two, her notion of how long she was going to be gone with Bill differed greatly from the length of time that they actually spent together. She'd say three weeks and it'd be closer to six days. Therefore, I was thinking she'd need meds for a week or ten days but first I'd talk to Bill after he had his train tickets and get the real story.

She was also upset about being gone for three weeks and yet still having to pay rent on her apartment. She said, "I'm begging you to get me outta here."

"Ma, I've told you many times that you won't be able to live by yourself, no matter what you think you're capable of. It's safest for you to be here and I want you to be safe."

She sobbed a little bit and said, "Well, could you at least think about it?"

"I've thought about it lots of times, Ma."

Without missing a beat, she cheered up instantly and chirped, "Oh good. When am I getting out?"

"Huh? Ma, just because I've thought about it doesn't mean you're leaving. In fact, it's the opposite. I've thought about it at length, and you have to stay. It's the best place for you right now." It wasn't what she wanted to hear, but instantly her attention drifted off again and I dropped the subject.

The next day I talked to Bill about getting dates arranged for when he was going to come out and take Mom to Austin. He said, "Do you know that your mother can be quite exasperating?"

"Yep."

He said that every time he'd talk to her about Austin, she'd then call one of the granddaughters and then things would change and, in short, he didn't know what was going on. I said, "When you have a window of dates that'll work for you, give me a call and I'll call Austin and we'll get it worked out. We'll keep my mom out of it until you and I have it all arranged."

Later that week, my daughters and I went to have dinner with Ma. The waitress brought me a cup of ice that I could pour my can of soda into, and when I took a sip, I smelled cigarettes. Nasty. Apparently, the waitress was a smoker and I could smell her hands on my glass. The dry burger was awful, especially when washing it down with the cigarette flavored cola. I did it a few times but then didn't drink anything else for the remainder of the meal.

As we rode up in the elevator afterwards, I noticed the ever-present calendar of events taped up inside the elevator. It showed that they'd cancelled the Easter parade and Easter-egg-hunt that they had scheduled for the next day, due to the virus. Virus? Excuse me? I asked Ma and she said, "I guess there's some kind of stomach virus going around and about half the people in here have come down with it."

So then of course, I couldn't get the smell from the cigarette hands out of my nose and somehow it seemed like this smell also carried the stomach virus with it. Disgusting.

When we were talking in her room she said, "I haven't talked to Uncle John (her brother) in a long time."

I said, "Uncle John passed away several years ago, Ma."

She laughed and came right back with, "Then it's no wonder I haven't talked to him."

I laughed out loud! It was refreshing to see a portion of her former wittiness make an appearance. These instances, as with so many of her character traits, were becoming fewer and farther between. Two days later, I was at home and received a text from my brother Jim, telling me that he had just called Ma and found out that she was very sick and throwing up. I didn't call her right then, thinking that she needed to rest.

EASTER SUNDAY 2014

We were having guests over for a big lunch affair. I was planning to get Ma and bring her over to our house, but with the virus situation and her being sick, I was at a loss as to how to deal with it. I certainly didn't want to expose anyone to the virus that my mom was dealing with, but I also didn't want her to miss the Easter festivities. After hemming and hawing for an hour or two, I decided that I'd call her and see how she felt before I made any decisions that might result in at least one person hating me. She picked up the phone and I asked her how she was doing.

"Oh, I feel much better today honey, but they have the whole place on quarantine. I can't even leave the building and they're bringing my meals to my room. I'm locked in here for two more days." She took it in stride and didn't mention anything about coming over to our house for Easter. It would have been great to have her over, but under the circumstances, it worked out for the best. No one hated me that day (as far as I knew).

Two days later, one of my daughters came down with nausea followed by the stomach flu. Then my next daughter got it. Then Sandy. Then the first daughter got it again and, finally, me. All told we missed a total of eight school and/or work days. Did it all stem from the assisted living facility virus? Probably. Seems like it would have been a good idea for the management crew to put a sign on the OUTSIDE of the EXTERIOR door to inform people that there was a stomach virus dripping through the facility and it might be best to hold off on visiting until things settled down a bit. Maybe the manager could also ask the wait staff to wear gloves either when they smoked, or when they worked in the dining room, or both. The place, literally, had made us all sick.

Ma said that she tried to do a little reading in the ALF library while the place was in virus-mode, but it didn't work out. I don't know if it was due to not being able to read very well or because she lost interest easily; perhaps it was a combination. She had been an avid reader for as long as I could remember. Fifty-two years of National Geographic magazines, along with many Michener novels, were in the basement. There were many other bookshelves positioned throughout her house that contained photography books, travel books, novels, and numerous magazines. Several years prior, she had even compiled a list of many of the books she remembered reading over the years. But that was before.

The following week we were talking in her room and she was, as usual, continually up and down and looking on the desk, in a drawer, in her purse or wherever, to show me something, anything, that she could come up with. Just observing her tired me out. She usually couldn't find what she was looking for, at least not at first. She had three or four stacks of papers on her desk and they were falling all over the place. She said more than once, "I gotta get this mess cleaned up. Maybe tomorrow. I also want to get home and straighten up the photo mess."

Then, once again, as she did during nearly every visit, she mentioned the rips in her bedspread, "I've got to fix these tears. I tried the other day, but I didn't have the right needle to do it.

I'll just wait until I get home and then I'll fix it on the sewing machine."

"How about if I bring you the sewing machine up here, Ma?"

"NO!" She continued to refuse to have anything more brought to her room while I continued to ask her and see if she'd changed her mind.

Just before I left she said, "Honey, when you get older and if you need to go to a place like this, just call me at my house and you can come there and I'll take real good care of you."

"Thanks, Ma."

She still had moments of compassion for others but her dementia, which drove her farther and farther away from reality, was on the other side of the coin. What kind of a disease does this to a person? The things that most of us would logically understand were getting farther and farther away from her. For example, if you assumed that I'd be her present age if/when I received a dementia diagnosis (78), then that meant that at that time, she'd be 102. As I mentioned before, my mom always had a knack for numbers but this latest example of her drift from reality was disheartening to say the least. She was completely sincere with her comment about taking care of me and I was flabbergasted and touched that she said it. Brain trauma is not to be taken lightly.

She never once mentioned Bill or the trip to Austin.

When I next saw her, she mentioned that she had decided to go on the most recent scenic drive in the ALF bus, and had asked the bus driver to go by her house because they were in her neighborhood. She wanted everybody to see her house, which was easily understandable, but who knew anything about this bus driver? I mentioned to her that she might want to be careful about telling other people that her house was empty. These things would have been a non-issue prior to dementia. She was too street-savvy for that and had always had a solid understanding of home security matters. She kept a baseball bat under her bed and a pistol in her closet. Now though, she threw her hands up and said, "Whatever."

She also mentioned that a roofing company had called her and said that there was some kind of a problem going on in her neighborhood and that she should consider having her roof checked out. Her roof was less than two years old and there hadn't been any damaging weather events since then to cause any issues. She told them to call me, which they never did.

She was beginning to get more and more anxious when it came to incoming phone calls. If she saw a number on her caller ID, when someone called while she wasn't in her room, she obsessed over who it might have been. She threatened to get out her address list and check EVERY NUMBER on it to see if it was someone she knew. Now, this address list was formidable. It was at least fifteen typed pages long, with a small font, and single-spaced. Speaking of that, she wanted me to print out a couple copies of the list so that she could start working on a project she had in mind. She wanted to list all the phone numbers numerically. That way, whenever she saw a number on the caller ID, she could cross-reference it to this new list, which she was not even remotely capable of compiling. I brought her the printouts and she tried for a few days before the idea went away. It was certainly a great idea though, and I told her so.

MOTHER'S DAY 2014

I had plans for taking her out for lunch on Mother's Day. I worked on Sundays, but that wasn't a problem because my lunch schedule was generally flexible. It was snowing like crazy when I went to pick her up around eleven and from there we went to her favorite Mexican restaurant. Before she fully sat down at the table, she made her signature comment, "I'm not a very big eater, so I hope I can find something on the kid's menu."

"No problem Ma, there's an ala carte menu and you can pick something from there and that'll be just fine."

I showed her where the ala carte menu was, and she just stared at it for a couple minutes. Her eyes were looking towards the menu, but she wasn't reading anything. She said, "I don't know what any of this stuff is."

Now, my mom loved Mexican food and had enjoyed it for decades. No hot spices for her, thanks, but she ate all forms of Mexican food whenever she had the chance. It was, by far, her favorite ethnic food.

I read off a few of the items that I thought she'd like and then she seemed to snap out of it and happily announced that she'd like a shredded beef burrito. When the waitress came and asked for her order, Ma just looked at me helplessly and I quickly ordered the burrito for her. Her increased reluctance to talk with other people and her declining level of comfort in social situations was apparent. But it was Mother's Day and we weren't going to let a little thing like that stop us from chowing down on some great Mexican food!

We were eating and talking away, and when she was about two thirds of the way through her burrito, she set her fork down and commented on the bowl of refried bean dip. She asked me what it was, and I explained. She looked at it and said, "I don't think I could eat another bite."

It was clear that the partial burrito had done her in. However, she apparently forgot that she felt that way because, within thirty seconds of making that statement, she was polishing off the last third of the burrito. After that, she set her silverware down and exclaimed, "I can't eat another thing."

I said, "That's good Ma, because there's nothing left!"

She said, "Yes there is, there's this stuff over here." It was, at most, a tablespoon of shredded lettuce and pico de gallo.

A few days later I went and had breakfast with her. After that, she had a checkup appointment with her doctor. She wanted me to bring some stuff home from her room, but I explained that there wasn't time. She wanted to ask the doctor about her going home. I mentioned that it wasn't up to him, it was up to me. She didn't like that answer at all, but she forgot it quickly.

Everything went fine with her doctor and he told her that she looked good and she replied "Yes. I eat very well. I'm eating three meals a day."

I talked to the doc offline for a few minutes and he did seem to be pleased with her condition. I explained to Ma that she was doing so well because not only had she been eating three meals a day, but she'd also been taking her meds correctly and exercising regularly.

She threw her arms up, "Whatever."

During the exam, the doc asked her if she had done anything special for Mother's Day. She threw her arms up again and, with the most convincing look of poor-me that she could muster, said, "Nothin'."

I teased her, "Nothing? You mean you don't remember that I came over during a blizzard and took you to that nice Mexican restaurant? And I got you a nice card and flowers, too."

She said, "Oh yeah, I guess I do remember that."

Later in the week, Bill called with a window of time when he could make the trip to Colorado, pick up Ma, and take her down to Austin so that she could see her great grandbabies. She was still very excited about seeing her first great grandchildren. Who wouldn't be? Bill asked me to contact the granddaughters in Austin to see if the dates he had in mind would work for them. He wanted me to let them know that Ma and he weren't planning to stay in either of their houses. Instead, they would be staying with an old friend of his and they would come visit the babies once or twice for an hour or two. He wanted to make sure they knew that he and Mom weren't planning on invading their homes or monopolizing too much of their time.

I then texted one of the granddaughters and she let me know that the whole summer was pretty much wide open other than two weeks that were unavailable due to previous commitments. Neither of these weeks would interfere with Bill's plans, so things were starting to come together. I called Bill with the news and he told me he'd call me back after he'd made the reservations. He also said that he wanted to hear from my mom that she wanted him to come, but I assured him that she did because she had recently started talking about it again and she really wanted to see him, her granddaughters, and the babies.

Later in May, my second cousin Sue, also from Boulder, called and said that she wanted to come down and see my mom the next day and take her to lunch. She was bringing a cousin of hers from New York (another second cousin of mine, whom I'd never met). Sue and I had discussed it earlier in the week and I mentioned that she should call my mom on Saturday, just to confirm that she was on board with the lunch get-together.

Sue called me back on Saturday evening and said that she'd just talked to Ma and that Ma wanted to cancel the lunch because she just didn't feel well. This would typically have been out of character for Ma because she always enjoyed going out to eat. However, as I explained to my cousin, Mom was getting more and more uncomfortable with any type of social situation. I then called Ma and asked her what was up.

"I just don't feel up to it, honey."

"But Ma, you always say you want people to come and visit and now she's coming down and you say you don't want to. I don't understand?"

"I just don't feel right honey, but I guess we can go."

"Well, I don't know Ma, I think maybe I'll call Sue back and cancel. I don't want you to go somewhere where you're not comfortable. Remember though, I'll be there with you and can help you order your meal and all that stuff."

"That's okay then, we can go."

The next Sunday, the girls came down from Boulder, picked up Ma, and I left work and met them for lunch. As expected, Ma was barely able to enter into most of the conversation, but she did fine in a few spots. She had some of her facts confused but she also had several that were right on. In all fairness, I had some of my facts confused as well. We were discussing the cousin's families, a group with which I was only slightly familiar. Overall, I'd say that my mom had a good time and she was glad that she'd made the trip.

A few days later, my brother Tom arrived from Thailand. He had originally planned to come and help sort through Ma's personal items and to help with preparing her house for sale. A couple months earlier though, he decided that he would come and stay indefinitely (he's retired). This way, Ma could live in her house and Tom would stay with her. I had told very few people about this because I didn't want Mom to find out too soon. If something went wrong with Tom's plans, she'd have been distraught and heartbroken and, although she'd likely forget about it, I didn't want to put her through the sadness.

Tom spent the night at my house and the next day we went and surprised Ma, which was hard to do because Tom's four inches taller than me and there wasn't any way that I could conceal him. She recognized him but was a bit out of sorts as we took her to lunch. I had contacted the medicine techs at the ALF, and they set us up with enough meds to last at least a week with the promise that they could continue with refills as necessary. At lunch, Ma was as nervous and anxious as ever. She held her hands under the table and kneaded them continually when she wasn't eating. She had gone through the buffet and loaded a heaping amount of food on her plate and then, during the meal, she once again remembered that she wasn't a big eater and instantly stopped eating. She wanted to know the location of the restaurant we were at, but she couldn't really grasp it even though it was in an area that she knew quite well. She asked, "What street are we on? What cross streets are we near?"

Tom took her home and started settling in. He called me later that night and said that Ma asked him to call me and PLEASE get the travel arrangements set up with Bill so that they could go down to Austin on their trip. I explained that I'd already done that and was just waiting to hear from Bill once he purchased the tickets.

I also explained to Tom that prior to Ma's stay in the mental hospital, she'd had a few DISASTROUS trips. Our poor mom had all these thoughts and ideas about what she wanted to do, because she'd always done them, but she couldn't do them anymore and everybody knew it but her, or at least that's how it seemed. Living in this false reality, while refusing to accept her current situation, was what had led to so much of her unhappiness while in assisted living. I must admit that I'm not so sure that I would do any differently were I in her shoes. It's easily understandable why she would act this way, because her actions were due to dementia as opposed to a conscious, logical decision on her part. I found myself respecting her refusal to give up but at the same time it pained me to see her suffering. If only she could have understood

SUMMER 2014

OPTIMISTIC, ANXIOUS, AND APPREHENSIVE

Tom was in-country for two days when he called from Ma's house and only had a few minutes to talk because the cell phone was a piece of junk. He was quite sure and firm in his beliefs that she was ready to come home for good and that we should give the thirty days written notice to the assisted living facility, ASAP. I was still apprehensive and felt that she wouldn't be able to deal with being at home or, just as bad, that Tom would realize that it was too much for him to handle and that we'd have to move her back into assisted living. If she had to go back to assisted living a year or two down the road, she'd be so far gone that it probably wouldn't be a big deal but if it was in the next six months or so, it would be quite confusing for her. He was optimistic, she was anxious, and I was apprehensive.

Later that day, they came to my house and she immediately headed for the couch and curled up into the fetal position. I hadn't seen her do that lately, but she hadn't been over in a little while so I wasn't sure what was up, although it seemed like she wasn't doing well. Tom and I went right to work and found out the scoop on getting her a pay-as-you-go cellphone plan and a reconditioned flip phone. Tom had already scheduled the installation of cable TV, a landline for the house phone and internet connectivity.

Tom mentioned that he had taken Mom to the YMCA because she wanted to go to a water aerobics class and then swim a couple lengths. She had never been overly fond of the water, but she had done water aerobics off and on for several years. When she was in assisted living, she never mentioned anything about going to the YMCA. Now that Tom was in town, she was perking up a bit.

Tom and I were in my bedroom office and Tom continued with more talk about how they had spent their day. After the swimming pool, they'd gone out to lunch and Ma was very talkative and had a great time. These types of events gave Tom and me a slight glimmer of hope while at the same time we knew that it was false hope. Regardless, it was always nice to catch these fleeting glimpses of her former self. Eventually, she came into the room where Tom and I were talking, to announce that, "We can go anytime, honey."

She was extremely anxious and uncomfortable and still wasn't doing very well. She may have just been tired because she went right back to the couch and lay down. That's when I typed up a two sentence, "notice to terminate the agreement" letter, for the ALF. I walked out to the front room, handed it to her, and asked her to read it and then sign it at the bottom. She stared at it for a couple minutes and I finally broke the ice, "Ma, can I help you with it?"

She said, "What is it?

"It's your get out of jail card!"

With that, she signed it right away. After this brief episode, I forgot how nice her day went and was quite worried about her, once again. She had stared the same way at the Mexican restaurant menu on Mother's Day, with zero comprehension. Neither of these were even slightly complicated items (unless you have dementia), yet she could NOT understand them. As mentioned previously, she had been an avid, lifelong reader but not anymore, man. Not anymore.

The next week, I called her granddaughter (my niece), in Austin and verified the dates that Bill and Ma would be there. She said the dates were fine and that she'd let her sister know. I offered the caveat that, "These plans can change at any time."

I swear, I wasn't off the phone for five minutes and Tom called, "Ma wanted me to call you and ask you to call Bill and cancel his trip to here and to Austin."

Uh, what? Isn't she the one who just encouraged me to call Bill the other day and cement the plans? Didn't I just tell Bill that he didn't need to talk to her because I was sure she wanted to go? Oh no! There was nothing to do except call Bill right away. He was maybe a little surprised, but not too much. He said, "That's why I wanted to hear her say that she wanted me to come out."

Ouch. I felt like a real idiot when he said that. Luckily, Bill had experience with dementia (his ex-wife), and he's very wise and understanding, so he seemed to take it in stride. He assured me that he was not mad and that he was only concerned about Ma. He stated that as long as it was in the summertime, he could drive from California in his own car, pick her up, and then drive on to Austin. If he did that, they wouldn't have to worry about train, bus, and other travel reservations (he doesn't like to fly). He's really a great guy and could surely have been more cantankerous. In fact, he wasn't cantankerous at all. I was off the hook!

On Ma's first night living back at her house after we moved her out of assisted living, she, Tom, and I were standing out in the front yard and it was pitch black. I was so happy for her and that she was finally able to come home. Prior to Tom announcing his plans to stay, I never thought she'd live at home again. She looked up in the sky and said, "There's only one star in the sky. Either that or it's an airplane that's stuck."

We went in the house and talked over how we were going to deal with the med's and get them switched to home delivery. Ma said she didn't want the pills in the blister packs, because it was hard for her to remove the pills from the packaging. I said that Tom would get them out for her. She said, "I know, but I'm talking about after Tom's not here anymore."

We let it go at that.

Within two weeks after Tom arrived, Ma was eating freshly prepared meals every day. Tom is a vegan and he puts great emphasis on eating fresh, organic food. And Ma, literally, ate it up. She was chowing down every day, every meal, and she started to gain weight. From June through September they were on the go, eating healthy and enjoying a quality of life that she never would have had if it wasn't for Tom.

He frequently took her to dinner with various friends. They took several rides up into the mountains, just to go have lunch or stop at a little mountain store that Ma liked. She didn't always know where they were, but she enjoyed the outings just the same. Tom joined a meditation group and Ma went with him to a class more than once. He was extremely patient and an excellent caregiver, and his actions enabled us to continue to catch small glimpses of our mom's former self. At the same exact time though, her overall mental condition continued to decline. Her cognitive deterioration was an out-of-control train, yet physically, things were looking up, or at least holding their own. Her blood pressure had stabilized nicely and, along with her weight gain, she was doing quite well.

Except she started to forget who we were.

Now, in all fairness, I sometimes call my two daughters by the other one's name. It happens. That's not what I'm talking about here. One night I was visiting with her and she was telling me about how Bill had come across a bunch of literature about Thailand. She said, "I told him that he needs to send that to John right away."

I said, "Ma, I'm John. I live here in Colorado. I think Bill should probably send that stuff to Tom because he's the one who lives in Thailand."

"No he's not!"

"Sure he is, Ma. I'm right here in front of you, right now. Try to remember."

Then she finally remembered, and things straightened out in her mind, but just for a little while. I wasn't surprised that she was starting to forget who we were, but that didn't help to lessen the blow. I had heard about this from several people who'd had the same experience. It's not pleasant.

One night, Tom brought Ma and we all met at the high school where my oldest daughter was participating in an orchestra concert. Ma always looked forward to these outings but hadn't mentioned it in quite some time. She clapped along and tapped her feet with her eyes closed, gently swaying back and forth with the beautiful music, which she loved to do. Two hours after the concert, Tom called to tell me that Ma had forgotten that she had gone to the concert earlier in the evening. She also didn't remember where her stereo was located. When she finally tracked the stereo down, she was surprised to discover that there was a piano in the same room. She always loved this little room, which she used to call The Conservatory.

> The next evening all of us went for drinks at a club near my house. It was during happy hour and there was a woman playing requests on a baby grand piano. Mom was having a great day and, after asking us to order her a glass of white zinfandel, she then asked the piano player to play one of her favorite old Irish songs. When the awesome piano player began to play, Ma closed her eyes and instantly went somewhere else in her mind. I don't know exactly what she was thinking about, but I'm quite sure that she was envisioning somewhere where she felt safe and happy. Suddenly, she was a younger version of her current self, someone who loved a glass of white zin and a favorite tune on the piano. There wasn't a dry eye in our group, and not a word was spoken, as we watched while she gently smiled and swayed with the music, just as she'd done at the orchestra concert the previous evening. It was quite touching and beautiful to see her respond in this way to the profound power of music.

In mid-September, we were talking about Bill and she said that she knew another Bill, but she couldn't remember his last name no matter how hard she tried.

THE TWO BILLS

One day, Ma said, "I talked to Bill Atkinson today and asked him if he knew who this other Bill was. He said that he didn't."

Naturally, I had always known Bill's last name, but she had never mentioned it when referring to him in the past. Ever. She always referred to him as Bill. I told her, "That's because there isn't another Bill, Ma. The only Bill you've known for a long time is Bill Atkinson. They're one and the same. There's no other Bill in your life."

"But I just can't remember his last name," she said.

"That's because his last name is Atkinson, Ma. There is no other Bill and you're just a little confused, that's all."

"Whatever."

The next week Tom, Ma, and I were in her front room and she was talking about the handmade end table next to her couch. She wanted to know about it, so I explained that our brother Jim had made it for her several years earlier. She remembered that, but what she couldn't recall is what happened to the other one! We explained that there never was another one in her house because Jim had only made one. She persisted for several days and Tom and I deduced that the second table must have been located in the front room of the second Bill.

This went on for a couple months and, as with many things of this nature, Tom and I learned to go with it. Sometimes we'd try to change the subject, but usually we would just go along. It was also during this time that Ma started to randomly speak using nonsensical words and sentences. She'd come into a room where Tom and I were talking and say, "I just checked my schedule….with the plants…and tomorrow's clock with the mayonnaise is upsetting." It was so hard to listen to this because she looked to be her normal self. In fact, she looked quite well. Unfortunately, by this time dementia was calling most of the shots. She increasingly had trouble getting dressed and needed more and more help with other tasks that we generally take for granted. My heart was breaking, and I'd look at her just wishing and hoping that she'd return to her former self of a couple years earlier, but that wasn't going to happen.

She and Tom were baking cookies one day and she called me on the phone and said, "Hi honey. I've got some yummy cookies for you guys and we want to come over for supper and bring these for desert."

"That'd be great, Ma, but give us an hour or two because we're right in the middle of something right now."

"Oh, okay, no problem. We'll just drop by Jim's house and drop some cookies off with him on the way to your place."

"Well, if you stop at Jim's, I'll see you in a few days because he lives in Illinois, Ma."

"He does not!"

Then I went into a lengthy explanation as to how many times she'd been at Jim's house and what it looked like and all that. It didn't matter though, so I changed the subject. She hadn't lost her touch with baking, that's for sure, and the cookies were excellent. Tom had been there to ensure that she included all the ingredients, and that they were fresh.

SOMEWHERE WHERE THINGS MADE SENSE

One night, I was sitting with her at her house and we were just talking away. She said, "I want to go home to Chicago or to Essex Lane."

I said, "Ma, we're at Essex Lane right now. You don't have a house in Chicago anymore. You sold the house in Oak Lawn a long time ago, remember?"

She didn't remember. She was so confused and scared, and it was very hard for her to deal with all these issues at the same time. Tom and I decided that "home" meant, to her, something like, "not here." Or maybe, "somewhere where things made sense." Something like that. The problem is that very little made sense to her and it didn't seem to matter where she was. She just wanted to go "home."

In mid-October, Tom phoned me one day and told me that Ma suddenly lost interest in eating. Just like that. This was very strange because, since she reached the point when she forgot that she "wasn't a big eater," she devoured any and all food put in her path.

Then she stopped.

I mean she STOPPED. It didn't appear to be a conscious decision on her part; it wasn't as if she decided to go on a hunger strike. It was like her body and/or mind had decided that enough was enough. One of the nurses explained that, with dementia, many times the person couldn't connect the dots that when something smelled good, that meant you should eat. Maybe the ol' taste buds weren't able to send signals to the brain any longer. Maybe, for some reason, at some level, she had given up?

Later in October, Tom called me at work and told me that Ma was very disoriented and out of sorts. She wanted to go see her doctor because, "Something just wasn't right." We decided that with the lack of eating and continual mental decline, along with her poor condition on this day, that it was time to get her to the hospital for bloodwork and to check other vital signs.

After a long day in the emergency room, Tom called to let me know that her sodium and potassium levels were quite low. I knew from prior experience with her that when the sodium and/or potassium levels went out of whack, it had a profound effect on her overall mood. She was also mildly dehydrated. Because of these issues, they admitted her to the hospital for a few days where they put her on an IV to bring the electrolyte and hydration levels back to normal.

I went to see her after work and she seemed to be doing fine, although she was very tired. It wasn't long before she started wandering, and when I came to see her two days later, she wasn't in the same private room. Before I got there, Tom told me that she was in a different room, a semi-private room. There was another patient at one end of the room, then there was a big curtain divider, and then there was Ma's bed.

There was also an additional person in the room. A "sitter." I had never heard this term before, in a hospital context, and the role of the sitter is just as it sounds. They worked in shifts and there was a sitter present 24/7. This was to prevent a patient from wandering off and ending up who-knows-where. Given Ma's history of previous escape attempts, this seemed like a good idea.

ALL THE KING'S HORSES AND ALL THE KING'S MEN

11/3/2014

They released Ma from the hospital because her electrolyte levels were within an acceptable range and she was feeling much better. On the way to Ma's house, they stopped and bought Tom some long underwear because it was starting to get colder outside, and his bones were used to the Thailand heat. Back at Ma's house, Tom had already moved his bedroom upstairs, right next to hers. It had previously been in the basement, right below Mom's bedroom and, because her wooden floors creaked like a haunted house, he could hear her when she moved around; now he wanted to keep an even closer eye on her. She was quite tired and fell asleep late in the evening, but then she'd get up every thirty minutes or so and wander around the house. She made sure that the doors were locked, and that the outdoor lights were on. Usually she'd use the bathroom and then wander around some more until Tom could finally persuade her to return to bed for the night.

11/4/2014

I was at work the next day and, at approximately noon, I received the following message from Tom:

"Hey John. Mom fell off the toilet in the middle of the night last night. We've been at the hospital for several hours now and she's still in quite a bit of pain. We're in the ER at the moment and they're looking at the pelvis, spine, and hip. Looks like a pelvis or a hip thing but the nurse isn't sure if it's a fracture or not. The phone reception in the ER is terrible so I'll come out every couple of hours and give you a call with an update. Ma's on pain meds so she's pretty blitzed out right now. I imagine we'll be in the ER for several more hours and then we'll probably get checked into a room. Talk to you in a little bit."

Oh no. OH NO!!

My work environment is far from private and in the ocean of cubicles that I was in, many ears would have been able to hear me if I lost it. I started to shake uncontrollably as my throat tightened and tears started to form. I couldn't control it and had to step outside for a breath of fresh air. I don't think it's necessary to expound on what it means in many cases when an elderly person breaks their hip or something equally traumatic.

I was able to reach Tom on the phone shortly after listening to his message because he, also, had just stepped outside for a breather. He explained about Ma's fall and said that he got to her very quickly after she fell but couldn't easily move her because she was in a lot of pain. He managed to get her back into her bed, which was a short distance away. Well, it would have been a short distance away if she didn't have a fractured pelvis. Tom is big and strong and had one heck of a time getting her the fifteen feet to her bed. He knew that she needed to go to the hospital just as surely as he knew that he couldn't get her there, so he called an ambulance. They had to put her in a soft stretcher of some sort as the floor plan of her house was such that a standard stretcher or gurney wouldn't fit. The ambulance then took her to the hospital ER, with Tom following behind.

I talked to him on the phone later in the day, after the doctors examined Ma, and it turned out that she had several fractures in her pelvis. Luckily, there was no bone displacement, so she didn't need surgery. This was good news, but it did mean that she couldn't stay in the hospital. Arrangements were made, and she was brought over to a rehabilitation center, where she could receive the help she needed to perform daily tasks such as using the bathroom and getting dressed.

I went over to the rehab center right after work and instantly didn't like the feel of the place. Tom felt the same way. The people we dealt with were fine at first, but we both knew it wasn't going to be a long-term stay. We'd find her another place. As it turned out, most of the staff there were nice, and very competent, but we soon encountered this one nasty little bulldog of a head nurse. And she was the one that put us over the edge. Tom, who spent much more time there than I did, had absolutely no use for her because she was very abrasive and rough. A few days later, he told me that Ma had really needed to go to the restroom. Tom pleaded with the bulldog, but she just barely acknowledged him and said, "The floor nurses will take care of that." She was completely indifferent to Tom or Mom.

I went to see Ma the next day and as soon as I walked into her room, she spotted me. She was lying in bed and instantly threw her blanket aside and said, "Let's go."

Things were going great until she actually tried to move. You see, she planned to swing her legs over the side of the bed and hit the ground running because she forgot about her injury. Suddenly, she remembered it very quickly and let out a yell that brought the staff rushing in (except for the bulldog), full speed. They told me that they thought she might have fallen.

Whenever Ma needed to go to the bathroom or get up for any reason, it hurt her. She'd yell out sometimes. Tom and I would try to help but it was usually best if we just got out of the way and let the pros do their thing. And boy, they did. It typically took two of them to get her into her wheelchair. Then off to the bathroom, up out of the chair, onto the toilet, back into the chair and then back into bed. Poor Ma was so confused and hurting that we could barely stand it, but what could we do?

She still ate little or nothing.

11/6/14

I had lunch with my kids and Ma at the rehab center cafeteria and I chose a nice little table next to a window because she loved to sit in the sun. I had secretly ordered fish for her, because that had always been one of her favorites and I thought she'd enjoy the surprise. As I was feeding her (correction - trying to feed her), I gave her the, "You must eat if you wanna get stronger, so you can do physical therapy, so you can walk, so you can leave" scenario. I cut the fish into bite-size pieces, but she didn't even attempt to eat it on her own. I put a piece on a fork and held it up by her mouth, but she wouldn't eat it that way either. Instead, she just smiled and laughed. It was as if she felt that she was onto my game and she wasn't going to let me get away with anything because she saw right through my plan. This was in no way a defiant gesture on her part. It was as if she was looking at it as kind of a joke because she couldn't comprehend the seriousness of not eating. She just wouldn't eat regularly, no matter what any of us did.

Once she became a resident at the rehab center, she didn't answer the phone or make phone calls anymore. If Tom or I dialed someone, and then handed the phone to her, she'd usually talk for a few minutes. Prior to this she'd make or receive quite a few phone calls on a regular basis. Not anymore. She also didn't bring up the subjects of driving or traveling. The saddest part of this was realizing that the last little bits of her personality were either going away or already gone. In addition to phone calls, driving, and traveling, we also said goodbye to any mention of her going home, her house, sewing, baking, water aerobics, reading, photography, shopping, sunbathing, gardening, or walking – because these parts of her, and many others, were gone. Most of these traits had been slowly disappearing, but after the broken hip it was as if she entered a new dimension.

She did pick up a new habit, though. She started to say "hurry," "hurry up," or "let's go," on a regular basis.

My mom told me several times when I was a kid about how her dad frequently used the phrase "Let's go, Ma," when he was out somewhere with my grandma and the family, and he was ready to go home. When I was sixteen years old, her dad passed away. It came to the point during the funeral service when most of the crowd had passed by the casket and said their goodbyes. Before the final closing of the casket, my grandmother, her four kids and their spouses, and several of us grandkids were there to say our last goodbyes to our beloved papa; it was so tender and touching that it still affects me some forty-two years later. My grandma was standing over papa as he lay in the casket. Her whole body trembled as she gently touched his head and face

with her shaking hands saying, "Bye papa, bye papa." After several minutes of this, when the rest of us had said our goodbyes for the last time, my mom put her arm around my grandma's shoulders and said quietly, "Let's go, Ma. Let's go."

Before she fell and entered rehab, my mom's conversational ability was declining. But once she entered rehab, her regular speech patterns ended. Just like that. As I mentioned earlier, she had difficulty forming coherent sentences at times, yet she was still able to talk with Tom and me frequently. Some of these conversations were reasonably lucid, and when they weren't, we had learned to interpret not what she said, but what she meant. The learning curve was steep but, at a minimum, we were usually able to understand what she was talking about, most of the time.

Another development that arose at this time was our accepting that she would never be able to live at home again. Ever. Tom, bless his heart, had reached the limit of his abilities. It was much easier to arrive at this decision now that it had become very apparent that she needed to be around professionals at all times. The emotional effect this had on Tom and me? Not so easy.

When I initially put her in assisted living, prior to Tom's arrival, I didn't think then that she'd ever be able to live on her own again. I suppose there had been a glimmer of hope that maybe, somehow, something would change and she'd be able to return home. As it turned out, this did happen when Tom landed and became her caretaker. But this time it was different. This time there was a finality to it that wasn't there the first time. This time it was cast in stone, and it hurt.

She wasn't very interested in helping her cause when she was in physical therapy at the rehab center. She had previously acted this same way following her back surgery; it hurt her to move and she just couldn't get much beyond that. Gradually, as the pain subsided, she joined in and started to show minor improvement. After two weeks she could walk without a walker if she felt like it, although she preferred to have someone push her in a wheelchair.

During her stay at the rehab center, Tom and I both received several phone calls from the staff. Sometimes they'd call and say that she was being cooperative (or uncooperative) when it came time for her physical therapy. Sometimes the call was due to her lack of eating. On one occasion, the nurse called me and said that Ma had pulled all the bedding off her bed, spread it out on the floor, laid down and went to sleep. They didn't know what to do. I thought about it and said, "I guess she can't fall off the floor. Let's just go ahead and leave her there as long as she's in a safe spot."

And that's what they did.

11/14/2014

As I mentioned above, shortly after Ma entered the rehab facility, we decided that we'd be moving her to another. Tom did quite a bit of checking around and found a location that we both agreed was the place to go. He made the arrangements and the transfer took place. The difference in care was remarkable. We didn't encounter any bulldogs there, just hawks, and they kept a very close eye on Ma; not every second of course, but they were very attentive. As with assisted living, the hospital, and now rehab, Tom and I showed up at all different times so that we could observe what was going on across all the different shifts and personnel. I highly recommend this as a way to check on the care facility in question. It's solid advice that an old friend recommended to me, and now I'm recommending it to you. Try to break up your schedule so that your arrival time isn't predictable. Not every single time, but do it frequently.

At this stage my mom was, for the most part, oblivious to what was going on. I don't recall her making any comments about where she was or why she had to move. Previously, this would have gone against her grain in a big way and, at a minimum, she would have demanded a full dissertation explaining the situation, most likely followed by her full rebuttal.

The lack of interest in eating continued, along with the expected weight loss. Her mental state was in serious freefall as she rapidly traveled downhill. She started to sleep more, except at night, and it was getting more and more typical of her to sleep for a portion of the time when I was there to visit. Consequently, I came to know the staff and a few of the residents quite well.

There was Bill. "Wild Bill," we called him. Several months earlier he had fallen and broken his right hip. He did his time in rehab and recovered. Then he went home, fell, and broke his left hip. Bill had advanced dementia, was a loose cannon, and obviously didn't care to be in a wheelchair. There was no doubt that he had plenty of spunk. Sometimes he'd get out of his wheelchair and try to make a break for it. On one such occasion, three or four CNAs came out of the woodwork as they maneuvered themselves to keep him from falling as well as to block his exit. At other times, I'd see him when he was generally calm, and I'd say "Hi," or "Hey Bill."

He'd give me the once over, think on it, and then say, "Howdy." One time he called me John Wayne.

Then there was Betty. She was just the loveliest elderly lady with a sweet voice and kindly manner. Unfortunately, she couldn't open her right hand. You see, Betty had suffered a stroke and, although her mind was quite sharp, her right arm and hand were still paying the price. I'd always tell her that the color in her fingers looked great and that she'd be grabbing an apple in no time. She'd then give me a great big smile. I don't know how much this helped her, but it helped to keep me from feeling so sad.

Let's not forget Sylvia Lee. Sylvia Lee was deep into dementia, yet she would have moments of relative clarity and we could have a somewhat normal conversation. At other times, she was gone. Once, I walked into the dining area on the way to Ma's room and Sylvia Lee was sitting at a table, all by herself. On the table in front of her was a large pile of bloody tissues. I went over to check on her and asked if she was okay. She couldn't talk that day, so I went and let the nurse know about the bloody nose. The nurse told me that her nose wouldn't bleed so badly if she'd just quit picking it. I found out that it wasn't unusual for a dementia patient to have any number of nervous tics, some of which could cause them harm.

On another visit, I saw Sylvia Lee and she had a large bruise that covered the whole right side of her face, along with her right arm. The bruises formed because she had fallen. I talked to the nurse and she said that people fell there all the time. This initially took me by surprise but, after she explained it, I understood. Even with the nurses, CNAs, RNAs (Restorative Nursing Assistants - a CNA with additional education/training), and caregivers, every patient can't be continually watched, 24/7. It's not possible. I suppose this was at least partially balanced by the fact that, when a patient fell, there was help close by.

When I met Sylvia Lee for the first time, she was one of Ma's tablemates. She was talkative as heck. I introduced myself and asked for her name and, without hesitation she joyfully announced, "I don't know!"

A short time later, a nurse brought her a pill and called her Sylvia. Again, without hesitation, Sylvia Lee responded with, "Actually, it's Sylvia Lee."

Ma had many issues that concerned us, but we were especially concerned with her lack of eating. Tom brought some coconut oil and she'd sometimes have a spoonful or two. Sometimes she'd have a glass of Ensure. On rare occasions she'd eat a fourth of a sandwich or a couple small pieces of fruit, but these were minimal. She also drank very little and dehydration was a continual problem, along with constipation. The nurses also suspected, no less than five times in two months, that Mom had a urinary tract infection.

She also began to have problems with holding her head up completely, which may have been because she was so tired and weak. At times, her head would roll around for no apparent reason. She didn't care for being in bed and she spent much of her time sleeping, sometimes in the fetal position, in a recliner by the TV. The nurses got to the point where they preferred her in one of the recliners, which were located right outside of their office. That way they could keep a closer eye on her, especially at night. Because on most nights, she liked to roam around aimlessly. They call this "wandering." Wandering is a common event in the dementia ward, and she had also been doing this when she lived at her house with Tom. We heard about this condition while in the first assisted living facility, but it didn't apply to Ma at that time.

For whatever reason, she still liked to crawl around on the floor, then lie down and go to sleep. Many of her symptoms were textbook dementia behaviors, but the crawling around and sleeping on the floor was not something that the nurses had seen, or even heard of, before. She obviously felt comfortable there, so we all agreed that there was no reason to try and change her mind. Several times, when I'd go to see her in the evening, I'd arrive and head for the TV area. Some of the residents were sitting at the tables, eating a snack or doing a puzzle. The staff was buzzing around doing their thing. The dining room crew might be clearing off tables or cleaning up the kitchen. Still other residents were watching TV. And there was Ma, out cold, lying on the floor, in a safe location off to the side with a blanket and pillow. You get used to this kind of thing. Well, you get used to this kind of thing as much as you can, anyway. Even the strangest behaviors can begin to seem normal when you see them often enough, at least in this case. Even though these types of behaviors became the new normal, I frequently thought about just how far my mom had drifted away from her former self.

THANKSGIVING DAY 2014

Sandy, the kids, Tom, and I, went up to see Ma late in the morning. She didn't remember my youngest daughter. Overall she was in good spirits, but that only lasted for an hour or so and then she declined quickly. She wasn't aware that it was Thanksgiving or even what Thanksgiving was. We had already decided not to bring her over to the house because she wasn't eating, she didn't know what Thanksgiving was, and she seemed to do better if she stayed in one place because it was less confusing for her. It was hard on Tom and me though, that's for sure.

For many years, decades really, my mom and dad would host a large Thanksgiving get-together in Chicago for all the relatives. There were grandparents, aunts, uncles, cousins, sisters, brothers, and friends, the whole package. Attendees ranged in age from newborns to eighty-five years old. There was laughter and music across the board. One of my uncles played the piano and/or accordion, depending on the situation. Sometimes my grandfather would dance with my grandma in the living room, and boy could he move! There was usually a nice fire in the fireplace to warm things up.

The wonderful smells of the feast filled the air and you could feel the love that we all shared, unspoken as it usually was. It was great, great fun and provided lifelong memories for me and those in my extended family.

Not this year buddy, not this year. Tom and I knew it was probably Ma's last holiday season but, as was typical for us during this period, we'd kinda pretend that it wasn't happening. We had a few glasses of wine and talked over past Thanksgiving get-togethers. We talked about Mom and held on to our hope, but both of us clearly knew that it was a false hope. It's not that the odds were against her; the fact of the matter is that there were no odds at all. Luckily, there were several kids at our house, and we had a ball playing with them and teasing each other. The food was awesome and there were plenty of happy moments, but Ma was never far from our thoughts.

11/29/2014

I went to see Mom in the morning. When I first saw her in her room, she looked ABSOLUTELY HORRIBLE. I freaked out a little. She stood slouched over and her manic eyes were dancing around all over the place. Her eye sockets looked like they had dark makeup applied, except she wasn't wearing any. Her false teeth were out and her face was drawn something awful. It was hard to tell if her whole head was shaking or if it was just due to her restless eyes. Maybe it was both. Other than her eye sockets, she was flour white. I seriously thought about calling an ambulance because she looked so bad. I asked the nurse if anything had happened to her and she said that they'd taken an x-ray of her abdominal area because she frequently complained of having stomach pains. The x-ray showed a calcification of some sort, which the nurses described as a hardening inside the body due to calcium deposits.

Ma didn't really talk to me this day because it was too hard for her. We went over to the dining area and she laid her head down, right on the table. I rubbed her shoulders and back, and when she lifted her head up, I asked her how she was feeling. She was barely able to squeeze out a weak whisper of, "Let's go." Then she laid her head back down. It's incredible what the mind holds on to until the end. She still wanted to "go." I called Tom and let him know how bad she was doing.

Several hours later, after I'd gone home, Tom was with Ma. I answered my ringing phone and it was Ma, saying, "What're you doin', honey?"

"I'm doing laundry Ma, what are you doing?"

"Oh, Tom and I are just here at the place."

She had rallied and was cheerful, lucid, and sweet as could be. She went on and asked about how school was going for the kids. She told me how she'd just talked to Aunt Mary on the phone. She was laughing and having fun with our conversation and thought that she'd start on a new jigsaw puzzle. The change from earlier in the day was incredible. I guess, on this day anyway, she just wasn't a morning person. Maybe when I was there earlier, she had just gotten up on the wrong side of the floor?

12/2/2014

Tom called me at work in the afternoon to tell me that Ma had been throwing up a green bile-type substance during the day.

The nurses and doctor suspected dehydration and decided that they'd put her on an IV. Tom said she'd been in the fetal position and out of sorts all day. He called me just before he went home and said that Ma was sleeping in one of the recliners in the TV area. A few hours later, I went to see her after work and she wasn't in the recliner. I went into her room and as I passed by the open bathroom door, I caught a glimpse of her on the toilet, naked. I quickly turned away and pretended that, "I saw nothin'."

I waited for her in a chair by the bed and discovered she had pulled out her IV needle and it was lying on the floor. She came out of the bathroom and started into Ruth's portion of their shared room when I stopped her and said that Ruth would probably enjoy the company but would most likely prefer that her visitors were dressed. I went to her dresser and found a nightgown for her to wear. The nurses came in and felt bad because they hadn't noticed that Ma had yanked out the IV needle and was now up wandering around. She had a large discoloration on her arm, about six inches long, from when she forcefully removed the IV needle. After she lay back down on the bed, we talked quietly and darned if she didn't mention "the two Bills" again. At one point, while she was lying there quietly and thinking, I asked her what was going through her mind.

"I'm afraid," she said.

"What are you afraid of, Ma?"

"People coming in and hurting me."

I asked her who would do that, and she said, "Bernadette."

I knew of no Bernadette in her life and there were no Bernadette's on the staff.

I said, "I'm not going to let anybody hurt you, Ma, so you don't have to be afraid."

Early in the evening, my brother Jim arrived from Illinois. Tom and I had both let him know that he should come sooner rather than later. Later in the evening, Tom's wife, Mai, arrived from Thailand. Later in the evening still, the nurse decided to put the IV back in. In the early hours of the morning, Ma ripped it out.

12/3/2014

Jim, Tom, Mai, and I were with Ma for the better part of the day. Mom was manic, agitated, and frequently throwing up. Her arms and hands were out of control, rotating around in these unexplainable circles, all over the place. Then she'd count out, for no reason that we could decipher, 55...56...57. 98...99...100. Then she'd yell out, "Call the doctor! Hurry. Hurry!"

She repeated this cycle five more times, and then five more. Tom asked her, "Why do we have to hurry, Ma?"

"Because I said so," she said, and that was that. Just a tiny bit of her lifelong feistiness was still hanging on. Given her current condition, the fact that she could still access that part of herself was quite remarkable.

The IV was back in place, secured by two rigid pieces of plastic that ran the length of her forearm. A variety of nervous tics had unexplainably assaulted her. She crossed her arms across her chest in an X pattern and rubbed her breasts, as if they were hurting badly. They eventually removed the IV because they were afraid that she'd pull it out again, possibly with dangerous consequences. She was so skinny that she could sit on a chair and bend her torso down such that she could touch the floor with the top of her head. This is not an exaggeration.

They did an X-Ray on her and we discovered that she had pneumonia, which led to a round of antibiotics. They also discovered that her potassium was low again, possibly due to a kidney issue. Late in the afternoon, they started her on nebulizer treatments to help with the pneumonia. A nebulizer is a small piece of medical equipment, consisting of an electric pump, controls, and a length of flexible tubing. Its function is to vaporize medicine for the patient to inhale, via a facemask in this case.

My youngest daughter needed a nebulizer for her frequent "breathing treatments" when she was a baby, and for a few years after that. The first time this appeared it was due to RSV (respiratory syncytial virus). She also had a rotavirus infection at the same time, which caused a bad case of diarrhea. She wasn't getting enough oxygen and she was also becoming dehydrated due to the diarrhea. This led us, her scared parents, to check her into the hospital, where she stayed for three days. Sandy stayed with her all night, and I was there all day. The hospital was a mess because the RSV had "gone viral" in Colorado Springs. There were three families crammed into the hospital room we were in, and this soon became the case in all the rooms. As the spread of the virus intensified, hospital beds soon lined the hallways because there was nowhere else to put them. Freaked out parents, including us, were everywhere. Our daughter recovered from this initial bout relatively quickly, which is more than I can say for Sandy and me – we were emotional wrecks. The breathing issues resurfaced several times over the next few years, but then they eventually went away for good. We purchased a nebulizer for home use (our daughter called it a "breathment treatment") and became quite adept at using it over the years. Now, because of my position as a member of the sandwich generation, I was

All the King's Horses and all the King's Men

experiencing the nebulizer again, but this time it was with my mom.

Ma was sitting on a chair in the TV area with the nebulizer mask on. I could hear her through the mask saying, "Let's go." .... "Let's go." .... "Let's go." On and on and on.

Her arms were still on autopilot and their frantic circling randomly continued. I sat in a chair facing her, off to the side and Jim was doing the same on the other side. Each of us had one of her hands as we tried to calm her down. Tom was behind her and had a hand on either side of her head while he talked calmly, also trying to settle her down. At one point she started leaning forward while bending down at the waist. She slowly kept going until she was lying on the floor. On my way down as I was assisting her, I looked up and there was Sylvia Lee, watching the proceedings from her wheelchair. I smiled at her and she started laughing hysterically. She wasn't laughing because of Ma's plight; she was laughing because dementia was bossing her around as well.

Eventually, during Ma's downward slide to the carpet, the nebulizer mask pulled away from her face. The vapor continued pulsing out of the mask that was still connected to its tubing but was now lying over the back of the chair. Ma was laid out all over the floor, the nebulizer mask was out-gassing, Ma was chanting, "Let's go," and Sylvia Lee was laughing like there was no tomorrow. The TV was blaring away (many residents were hard of hearing) and some of the folks were watching either it, or us. Two men had been working on a jigsaw puzzle, but now they were frozen in place, both of them staring in our direction and each holding a puzzle piece in their hand. The older upright piano was silent. Tom had played it on several occasions, but now was not the time. On top of the waist-level shelves where the jigsaw puzzles were kept, sat a coffee pot of, typically, cold coffee. People rarely drank it, which might have a lot to do with why the pot was unplugged and it was cold (I tried it once, and that was enough). I'm guessing it was old too, because, well, nobody drank it. Old and cold. The eight tables in the dining area contained one sole occupant, and that was an elderly woman, yelling for help. The cool, competent, incredible staff members were buzzing around, business as usual.

Jim, in the beginning stages of shock, and I, were on our hands and knees, right next to Ma's head and doing our best to comfort her, when I looked over at him and whispered, "Just another day on the dementia floor."

THE GOOD-LOOKING NUN - 12/4/2014

Ma was in much better shape today, although her stomach was bloated a bit, and she continued to complain about pain in her abdominal area. She went to the hospital emergency room late in the afternoon because of her bloated stomach. Tom and Mai followed the ambulance over to Penrose Hospital and waited for the results. The doctor concluded that the bloating was due to ascites, which is fluid buildup in the abdomen. They also discovered a wound of some sort on her liver.

While Tom and Mai were waiting for the completion of Ma's tests, they grabbed a cup of coffee and a snack as they tried to keep calm. They then wandered around the first floor of the large hospital, casually exploring. As they rounded a corner in the maze of hallways, they happened upon a large black and white photo on the wall. It was a photo of a nun, which in and of itself is nothing unusual, except for one thing. The nun looked like me.

> I didn't see the photo until two years later when Tom was in Colorado for a visit and we went to the hospital to see if we could find the photo of my alleged look-alike, which we did. When using our cell phone cameras, if we cropped the photo just right, effectively removing the nun's habit from the image, well, she looked very similar to me. I then stood next to the photo and Tom was taking a few snapshots of my doppelganger and me, when an ER nurse walked by and stopped in her tracks. She gave us a skeptical look as we struggled to restrain our laughter until we finally broke down and told her the story. This caused her to switch from a doubtful look to a more investigative gaze and it wasn't long before we were all laughing out loud. A janitor pushing his cart walked by, just in time to hear the explanation as to what we were doing, and he joined in too. Eventually, the nurse had to return to work, so we all said our goodbyes. She walked away laughing, and when she was ten feet away she turned around and said, "If you ever come to the ER here, you ask for nurse Rosie and I'll take good care of you. We'll pick right up where we left off!"
>
> So I've got that going for me.

At this time, we were looking for anything to smile or laugh about, which worked out well because almost everyone we told about this thought it was funny. In fact, almost everyone thought it was beyond funny. It was hilarious. Tom began to introduce me as, "My brother, the nun."

When it was time to leave the hospital and go back to rehab, Ma rode with Tom and Mai instead of in an ambulance. Hey, it was Christmas time! There were Christmas lights around town and Ma loved to look at them, while listening to Christmas music of course! Tom said that she really perked up while on this drive. She read every sign in sight, while singing along with the

Christmas music on the car stereo. I think maybe Tom knew that this was to be Ma's last joyride around town, but he never said as much to me. We all knew Mom was nearing the end, but maybe if we just kept reading the signs on the road, singing songs, and trying to get Mom to eat one more spoonful of apple sauce, somehow, some way, we might be able to save her.

She was back to rehab by bedtime, when the nurse explained to us that we had to decide if we wanted to go any further with Ma's stomach issues. My brothers and I discussed it at length and, due to the abundance of mental and general health issues that were occurring, we decided that no further exploration was necessary. Perhaps later we'd change our mind. Shortly after her return from the hospital, Ma started to fade quickly, and the hand rotation started again for no obvious reason. She said, "I don't know," very, very often, although, "Let's go," continued to be her mantra of choice.

In the midst of all this turmoil, she was still able to flash her nice smile occasionally. This, along with fleeting eye contact, was rapidly becoming her only form of communication with us. And these gestures were becoming fewer and farther between.

12/5/2014

Ma went into Ruth's section of their shared room again, naked, and took the false teeth from Ruth's bathroom counter. Ruth had been complaining that she wasn't comfortable with this arrangement and who could argue with that? The staff thought about moving my mom to another room and asked me what I thought. I told them that she'd probably just take her new roommate's teeth, so there probably wasn't any reason to move her.

She still wasn't eating, and this caused her to lose approximately three pounds every week. The jury was out on whether or not she was showing any improvement in physical or occupational therapy. In her case, physical therapy was the act of improving her strength, flexibility, and balance. Occupational therapy helped with everyday tasks such as going to the bathroom.

12/7/2014

The staff decided to move my mom to another room, which was a good thing in this case because it was a private room.

It was beautiful to watch how tenderly Jim took care of Ma as he took her for a walk in the wheelchair. Normally you'd picture Jim with a wrench in one hand and a power tool in the other. He was a great craftsman and could build or fix just about anything. But now, you could really see his tenderness shine through, beneath his tough, calloused hands. As they came back from their walk, Jim stopped and helped Ma with a jigsaw puzzle. Tom and I joined them, and we were all trying to help Mom, when suddenly our conversation turned to, "I need a brown piece for Bambi's ear." What? The jigsaw puzzle became our new focus for a few minutes as we tried to somehow maintain our sanity as the rest of our world fell to pieces with Mom's continual decline. It was extra painful for Jim because there was no getting around the fact that this would be the last time he'd see his mother. He was visibly shaken and out-of-sorts. Tom and I had more or less acclimated to this way of life but for Jim, or anybody else, coming in fresh was quite a shock. Quite a shock. Eventually, it was time to take him to the airport for his flight back to Chicago. Later, in the early evening, my two nieces arrived from Texas (Ma's granddaughters). Ma recognized them, and they had a nice visit for a half hour or so. Then she started to get cranky and loud in the dining area, yelling at Tom, "I don't WANT to eat!"

When he tried to help her walk she yelled, "I don't NEED any help!" This was such a contrast to her former self; as I mentioned previously, as far back as I could remember, I had rarely heard her yell.

It seemed likely that she possessed enough awareness to realize that she didn't want to appear helpless in any way in front of her granddaughters, and you couldn't blame her for that. It might have been that she was upset because new visitors were in town and she just didn't know how to deal with any of it. Hard to say.

12/8/2014

The granddaughters came up to visit with Ma again and this time they brought the babies, the identical twin daughters of the oldest granddaughter! My mom's first great-grandkids, and she was finally able to, "See those babies!"

Everybody was rested and in a good mood. Ma was all smiles and glowing with a skin color that I hadn't seen on her in months. She was happy! She wasn't able to talk much, but her recognition of her four special visitors was evident. This lasted for an hour or so before she began to fade and lose touch. For one brief hour though, she was a happy and proud great-grandmother and they were able to get several nice photos and have fun visiting. Her granddaughters, sad with the knowledge that this was the last time they would see their grandmother, had to leave for home the next day.

I went to see Ma after work the next night and she was really out of it. I asked her if she was in pain and she started rubbing her breasts like crazy and said, "My breasts burn."

I talked to the nurse and she said my mom hadn't been eating and she'd also been throwing up. She was also very restless, so I asked the nurse about an anti-anxiety pill, pain pill, or whatever she thought was best. She started with an anti-nausea pill, followed later by an anti-anxiety pill. I called Tom after I made it home and he told me that, earlier in the day, he had been cleaning up Ma's vomit and noticed that she had vomit on her ear. He asked her how that happened. Her reply? "It wasn't easy."

Now, you tell me, how could she possibly come up with a witty response like that, given her circumstances? She didn't eat and most of the time she couldn't talk. She had been a naked false-teeth-thief and yet she still managed to formulate these crafty words and deliver them with perfect timing. We couldn't explain it.

12/10/2014

Tom and I met with the pertinent staff to discuss the fact that our mom was no longer showing progress with physical therapy or occupational therapy. The therapists had discussed this amongst themselves and then explained to us that they could no longer say that she was improving. A requirement of Medicare made it necessary to document her status and her current status was, "not improving." This meant that she could no longer stay in the rehab unit on Medicare's dime. She would have to move to a private pay, non-Medicare assisted room, by Friday. We were very grateful for the short time that Medicare did pay for her care, as it surely helped with the financial side of things.

The staff told us that Ma had been crawling more and more. We never discovered if this was due to pain or to the dementia, or what. For whatever reason, she continued to prefer staying closer to the ground. Yet, when she was upright, walking didn't seem to cause her any problems, indicating that the fractured pelvis seemed to have healed nicely. She continued to have many bouts with her potassium levels, among other things, and the nurse informed us again that this could be due to kidney issues of some sort.

Her weight was down to ninety-six pounds.

Tom and I decided to start her out in the Memory Care area, the next level up from assisted living, although the nurse in our meeting felt that she belonged in Long Term Care, the highest level of care available at this facility. Tom and I thought we'd start with Memory Care and see how it went because she could always move to Long Term Care later if it became necessary. We went and looked at a few rooms in Memory Care and liked it, and the staff, very much. The sales lady, of course, showed us the larger/more expensive rooms first and didn't even mention a smaller/less expensive room. Luckily, Tom thought of it and we knew right away that the smaller room would be fine. It's best to watch these salespeople very closely. They may just be doing their jobs but, evidently, their job is to rent the highest priced room that they can. That's what we saw.

12/11/2014

We moved Ma's bed and dresser, from her house, into her new digs in the Memory Care unit. Déjà vu from October 2013 when

I first moved her into assisted living. The room that she had just vacated in the rehab unit was furnished, but this one wasn't, which meant that we also brought her rocking chair, large green teddy bear, and numerous fleece comforters, which she had previously made for many family members. Without question her favorite of these blankets was the Chicago Cubs model.

Although I grew up in a southwest suburb of Chicago, we were all diehard Cub's fans (the Cubs play at Wrigley Field, which is on the north side. The White Sox play on the south side). She would have been ecstatic if she had been around when the Cubs won the World Series in 2016. She would have joined me on my front porch, screaming at the top of my lungs when they clinched the final game. I'm sure of it.

It was obvious right away that there was much less staff in Memory Care. All the residents were dementia or Alzheimer's patients, in addition to the various physical problems that affected many of them.

In Rehab there were at least one, sometimes two, RNs and at least three CNAs. There were approximately fifteen residents, max.

In Memory Care, there were no RNs and no CNAs and just two caregivers (similar to a CNA but CNAs have an educational requirement to become CNAs, and caregivers don't). Here, also, there were approximately fifteen residents, max.

The caregivers were wonderful, but they were quite limited as to the decisions they could make on behalf of the patients. On one hand, the care level dropped tremendously and on the other, Ma's condition had worsened and kept declining. Perhaps we should have listened to the nurse in the meeting and went straight to Long Term Care?

I sat down with her for lunch and when we were finished (she had one spoonful of pudding) she yelled, "LETS GO!" at the dining room table. She, at times, was becoming increasingly loud and angry, although she didn't have enough strength to be violent.

For the last week or so, she had continued to become less and less talkative for whatever reason. And that went for talking to anybody. She also became more and more distant, even with Tom and me. You hear about these types of symptoms but, as in many cases, hearing about something is much different than going through the experience. I found myself having more and more difficulty concentrating at work and at home. I tried not to think about it, but I couldn't control this very well. At work, on several occasions, I'd have to go to a private area and have a mini breakdown. Sometimes, in the middle of the night, I'd wake up tossing and turning as I thought of my mom. I thought of things she did for me, for us.

Sometimes I thought of small things like talking with her on her screened back porch, shaded by the three gigantic maple trees in the back yard. A slight breeze was typical. We'd have a cup of tea and talk about traveling, fishing, the kids, Illinois, whatever subject we felt like talking about. As I mentioned previously, she didn't always care for small talk, but something about that back porch in the summer caused her to loosen up a bit.

Other times, I'd think of things that she had done that were major memories for me.

One summer, when I was eleven years old, I thought I'd become a paper boy and deliver newspapers in the morning. I knew other kids that did it, and I could see myself zipping down the street

on my bike, effortlessly tossing the papers with deadly accuracy, until all the papers were gone. Except it didn't work out that way. My bike wasn't the type that could easily handle a large cloth bag of newspapers. I was small and not very strong. I couldn't handle the load and the bike crashed several times, spilling the papers out all over the street. After a half hour of this, I was exhausted and the only paper that I'd delivered was the one that went to OUR house. I managed to limp my bike home, where my mom was getting ready for work. I was shaking and visibly upset when I blurted out, "Everything's going wrong, Ma."

She stopped what she was doing, right then, and headed towards the back door with one arm around my shoulders and said, "Let's go, honey."

We jumped in the VW beetle and went to where I'd left the bag of papers by the side of the road. After cramming them into the back seat, away we went with the list of addresses on my lap. My lack of strength was no longer a problem, which made it easier to notice my lack of accuracy, but we delivered every one of the papers that day.

This story and many, many others had been on my mind since this whole thing started and they were now becoming more and more frequent. There were also the increasing doubts I'd also had since the beginning: Was I a good enough son? Would my dad have approved of the way I was dealing with things? Should I have tried harder to keep her out of assisted living in the first place? Was she in the best facility we could find? What else could I have done? It was a very difficult part of my experience and had taken a cumulative toll on me. Through all of this, I'd come to understand that dementia was not only hard on the patient, but on everyone involved.

LET'S GO

12/14/2014

I stopped by after work to visit with Ma. When I walked in, she was sitting at a table in the dining area, which was a nice change but it had nothing to do with her eating anything. That just happened to be where she was sitting. She looked right at me but there was very little recognition. It's unclear if she knew who I was, but I sure didn't know who she was. At one glance, I could tell she was a different person than the one I'd seen just a few days earlier. I had an instant, reflexive thought that this was no longer my mom. She had changed. It was in the way she carried herself and the way she looked at me. I think she looked through me. Tears were slipping out of my eyes. I wasn't sobbing, but I couldn't stop them from flowing. I was also shaking and quickly sat down next to her before I lost my balance.

She had been changing for over a year now, but this was remarkably significant. She had degraded, exponentially, from our last meeting and I was able to arrive at these thoughts and feelings from a single glance. I knew right then, without question, that the last semblance of my mom's personality had completely vanished forever. And boy did it hit me hard as I sat there and digested these thoughts. Oddly, at the same time, she looked more aware and lucid. Unfortunately, this was a façade that was certainly unintentional on her part, and that became clear to me early in the visit.

I noticed that her socks were off. In general, she was not a bare-footer, so this was very unusual. Her socks were on the table and she was extremely interested in the wheels attached to the bottom of the table legs. A foot lever that operated the wheels pushed them down, which then made the table easier to move. I said hi to her and she said, "That was thirty-nine under there."

This was a version of the "numbers thing" that had recently become so prevalent. "Let's go," she said, "let's go."

We had seen many instances over the last few months where something completely unrelated to what we were talking about diverted her attention away from the conversation in progress. Sometimes she'd stop in mid-conversation, point, and ask, "What's that?"

It could be a star in the night sky. Maybe a spider web. Perhaps a jellybean. The point being that it would be something completely unrelated to what we were discussing. It seemed that her mind could still focus, albeit barely, but the direction in which it focused was randomly directed, at least from our frame of reference. The wheels under the table were a perfect example. I still find it remarkable enough to mention that, when she was inspecting the wheels underneath the table, she managed to keep her butt in the chair while bending completely under the table to touch the wheels, twice.

To reiterate, she was surprisingly lucid looking, but blatantly worse off in the mental department. As I mentioned previously, she had already started to forget who Tom and I were, but, at the same time, there were days when she knew us perfectly well. Now it was getting to the point where not only did she frequently not know us, but she didn't know that she didn't know us. This was one of those days.

There was a new lady resident at her table that kept repeating "My, my, my, my, my….." I never did learn her name.

Ma had one of those little plastic, kinda-kidney-shaped bowls that hospitals always have for you when you're a patient, out on the table. In it, she had a hairbrush, comb, and toothbrush. After an hour or so she decided to put her socks on. She then put the comb inside one of her socks, underneath her bare foot. I told her she might want to get the comb out of her sock so that it didn't hurt her foot. She tried, but then she crossed her legs and got confused as to which sock contained the comb. I told her it wasn't in the one sock and that she needed to uncross her legs and lift the other foot. She couldn't get the correct foot. Finally, I tried to get the comb out and I had the wrong foot on my first shot, too. It was as if she was a shell game expert and she had seen me coming from a mile away. Then she put the comb in the kidney bowl and tried to put the bowl on her foot, like a shoe.

Once we solved the footwear issues, we headed for her room and it was apparent that she was still walking much better and that the pain from the pelvic fracture seemed to have left for good. Of course, this also meant that she was now able to wander at will and it became necessary to keep a security bracelet on her so that if she tried to leave the area, an alarm would sound. She wanted to walk around but her strength had gone down tremendously and she wasn't able to walk very far. In her pre-dementia life, she always loved to go for a walk. Less than a year prior, she could easily walk three miles.

We finally made it to her room and shortly thereafter she received anti-nausea and other medications. Then she lifted her left foot while in the wheelchair and said, "This is 86. Let's go."

I asked her, "Is the other foot 85 or 87?'

"85," she said, "now let's go."

She started counting "85, 86, HURRY!"

Then she threw up. She vomited several times into the trashcan I placed between her legs and, in-between two of the vomiting sessions, she somehow managed to utter, "Let's go."

12/16/2014

I went to the ALF after work, talked to a caregiver on the way in, and heard that Ma was not having a good day. She was very restless and hollering almost non-stop. When I first arrived, I heard the normal sounds like the TVs blaring and people talking. Once I heard about Ma's condition, I focused my hearing and pretty soon I could hear her hollering. I was one hundred feet away and there were all kinds of other noises, but I could clearly hear her. "Hurry. Hurry. Hurry!" Louder, then quieter, then louder. It was constant, and it ripped my guts out. That was my mom yelling in there.

"Operator hurry. Hurry!"

I quickly moved to her room and when I walked in she could not cognitively recognize me when she briefly opened her eyes, which she then kept closed. It was as if someone, or something, had occupied her body, because this couldn't be my mom. I asked her if she hurt and she nodded yes, while keeping her eyes closed. I told her to touch where it hurt, and she instantly put her hand to the right side of her navel. I put my hand over hers and noticed that I was trembling. I was there for over three hours and she yelled out constantly.

Nonstop.

Usually, at least two of her limbs were rotating randomly in the air. Sometimes, when she was on her back, all four limbs were in the air and circling. Although she didn't seem to be aware that this was happening, it must have been extremely exhausting. She was out of control and I could not say or do anything that would calm her down or snap her out of this state. I thought that maybe if I sang to her it might help so I sang Rudolph the Red Nosed Reindeer three times, and this seemed to help her concentrate on my voice a little, but it really didn't change anything.

She'd lie on the floor, then get up and lie on the bed. At one point, I lay next to her on the bed and held her as I quietly wept. The caregiver came in and I said, "Ma, why don't you tell her how you used to drive up to Alaska by yourself and sleep in the car some nights. Tell her about the bears that you saw fishing in the river."

There was no response from her whatsoever as her erratic behavior continued. I asked the caregiver, "What causes her to act like this?"

Without hesitation she said, "Pain."

Period.

I asked the caregiver what I needed to do to help my mom and she said that their hands were tied and that they were required to follow the doctor's orders. Understandably so, but something had to be done. I then called the hospice group (Tom had just gone through the hospice admittance forms that very morning). The hospice nurse I talked to said that she'd make some medication changes and that if Ma didn't get better in an hour or two then she would come in to be with her. As it turned out, Barb, the hospice nurse, came in at eleven that night and was there until four in the morning. Hospice is truly a wonderful, wonderful service.

I heard after the fact that Ma became much worse after I left, which seemed to indicate that she still appeared to have some recognition of me. I explained to Barb that pain elimination was the immediate, primary concern, regardless of the medication required because Ma was clearly suffering very badly. My mind was racing at 100 miles per hour, as was my heart, and I had a tennis ball in my throat. It was the worse yet as I realized that this was another completely new level of "my mom is gone, and she isn't coming back."

For the next two days Tom and Mai were with Mom all day and into the evening. I talked to Tom frequently and knew that Ma was resting more and more because the pain medication helped to settle her down.

12/19/2014

When I first arrived, Ma was lying in bed and talking quietly: "Hurry, hurry, hurry. 38…39… 45. Hurry operator. 37…68…51. Hurry."

She sounded so terribly weak and was overall much quieter and calmer then she had been. Mentally, she was completely gone. She'd look at me then fall asleep while I sat there with my eyes full of tears. I found out that she'd had a large bowel movement, which seemed to have removed the fist-sized lump in her abdominal region. She was physically drained and completely exhausted.

She wasn't visibly suffering though, and she continued to sleep. Every five or ten minutes she'd quietly say a few words while keeping her eyes closed. When she did wake up, she wanted to leave. Later in the afternoon, as the sun was going down, everything in the room was cast in a dim gray, which added to the surreal surroundings. I was sitting next to her on the bed, comforting her with my arm around her shoulders, when she abruptly stood up, walked around the rocking chair that was next to the bed and, instead of trying to leave the room, turned around and kinda did a slow-motion fall back towards the bed. I was right there to catch her and lay her back down. She had given it everything she had and made it about eight feet. Her poor, damaged mind was barely able to make promises that her extremely weakened body could no longer deliver. It was awful. Just plain awful.

"Hurry...Operator....We haveta set the clock."

I told her that I did set the clock right after she told me about it, so she could now put her arm down (it was circling in space) and rest. And, much to my amazement, she laid her arm down and fell fast asleep. This visit, as with so many others, just devastated me. My eyes and cheeks were red in conjunction with my swollen throat. I was shaking and my pulse rate was out of control.

12/20/2014

Sandy and a friend of hers went to visit with Ma. I mentioned to Sandy that she needed to steel herself, as Ma had degraded quite a bit in the week or so since she'd last seen her. Sandy told me later that she had steeled herself, but not enough. When they got to Ma's room, Ma was sitting inside her opened suitcase, which was half in the closet and half out. She pointed towards the door and kept repeating, "Let's go."

They held her, talked, and all things considered, had a generally nice visit. Sandy lost it several times while there and again on the way home.

It seemed obvious that Ma was very close to the end, and it had for the last several weeks. Tom and I would discuss how we didn't think Mom would make it to the New Year. Then we'd say she probably wouldn't make it to Christmas. Then the next day we'd talk about making sure we had enough cash in her checking account to pay the next month's bills. We were all out of control.

12/21/2014

I was on vacation this week, so instead of working on Sunday as usual, I was home. I went over to see Ma mid-morning. I talked to the caregiver on the way in and she told me that Ma had been having a good night and morning, and that she was resting comfortably.

I went into her room and there she was, curled up under a blanket, sleeping quietly. She looked like an old, little girl. I kissed her on the cheek and told her I loved her and that everything was okay. She stirred a little, but I didn't want to wake her because she surely needed to rest. I just pulled a chair up right next to the bed and watched over her. Every so often I'd rearrange the blanket on her because it would sometimes get out of place when she changed position. At times, I half sat/half laid down in the bed with her. I'd put my arm around her head and, again, tell her I loved her and that everything was okay. When I touched her shoulders or rubbed her back, I could feel the bones that were protruding because she'd lost so much weight. It was heartbreaking.

After a few hours, I let her be so that she could continue to sleep. She never said a word while I was there.

12/22/2014

This was a Monday, and at approximately ten a.m., Tom called and told me that he'd heard from the hospice nurse and found out that they had done an assessment of Ma's condition that morning. It turned out that she had a condition on her feet called mottling. This referred to her having mottled, or blotchy, skin, which was due to decreased circulation. They also told Tom that Ma's extreme restlessness, especially what I had seen the previous Tuesday, was due to another condition called terminal agitation. In this context, "terminal" ranked right up there with final, fatal, and end of the line. In short, it wasn't good news. In fact, it was horrible news and even though we knew her condition was steadily deteriorating, there was now no denying that she was near the end.

And by this I mean, THE END.

They said it could be hours, or maybe days, nobody knew for sure. The only thing that was certain was that Ma's end was imminent. After hearing this, I wanted to get over there as soon as Sandy and the kids got home so that Sandy could go with me. I texted her and let her know what was going on and she said she'd be home shortly.

When Sandy showed up, I talked to the kids and told them that their gramma was in bad shape and that they could come see her with us if they wanted to. They were afraid to go, and I understood, so Sandy and I grabbed our coats and headed out the door. My phone had been on a table and before I put it into my pocket, I noticed that I'd had a call at 12:15. I guessed that I'd been in the shower and never heard the ring. There was a voicemail from Tom. Wait a minute.... I'd just talked to him less than two hours ago. Why would he be calling me back so soon? I called him right away on his home phone, but there was no answer. He had planned on going to see Ma at 2:00 so he should've still been home.

Uh oh.

My heart was racing and I felt weak. I was having trouble breathing. My dizziness made it hard to stand correctly, so I sat down as I continued freaking out. I think I knew......

I called Tom on his cell phone. He started the conversation with, "John, I....." and he went silent because that was all he could get out. He couldn't manage anything else at the time.

I was glad I was sitting down because my world collapsed and I was barely able to force out one word, "No."

"Yeah. Mom passed away about twelve o'clock. We're on our way over there right now," he said.

I broke down and wasn't able to talk very well, so I told Tom we were on our way. First, I wanted to go and tell the kids. My oldest daughter was on her bed, drawing, and I said her name and she saw my face and said, "What's wrong, Dad?"

I wasn't capable of smoothing things over for her and I was lucky to squeak out, "Gramma just died honey."

She came over and gave me a big hug and I told her we needed to leave because the nurse was going to meet us at one thirty. Then I went into the bathroom, where my youngest daughter was in the shower, and I called her name. She peeked around the shower curtain and saw my face and I said, "Gramma just died honey."

Let's Go

She instantly started crying and knelt down in the bathtub. I reached in, rubbed her back and explained why we needed to leave.

We arrived and entered Ma's room and Tom, Mai, and a nurse were in there already. Tom and I had a big hug and everyone was crying. Ma was on her back in the bed and she was definitely no longer with us. I've been around deceased people before and I have no idea if it's possible to get used to it. What I do know is that I wasn't used to it. There was my beautiful mother, in her characteristic green and turquoise clothing, and she was gone. God it hurt. A deep, cut-you-to-the-bone kinda hurt. Part of me was glad, because she didn't have to endure living inside a body that she no longer wanted. But this wasn't stronger than the fact that I'd just lost my mom, forever.

I hugged her and just kept rubbing her left shoulder. I wasn't able to say much. She was still warm to the touch and her shoulder was generally soft. She had reasonable color in her face, but it was starting to leave her. We all talked a little here and shared a memory there, but the exact goings on are generally lost. After a time, we had to talk to a woman about what funeral home we'd like to use, and all the logistics that go along with that.

We were there about two hours when the funeral home employee showed up. Tom and I helped him wrap Ma in a sheet and then a protective top cloth. We then said our last goodbyes to her face before we both covered it up with the sheet and the cloth. We were crying our eyes out as we gently covered her face and said, "G'bye, Ma."

All three of us then lifted her onto the stretcher. Then we wheeled her out through the common area and there was a trivia game going on with the residents, led by a caregiver, who called out in her cheerful voice, "Who can name one Marilyn Monroe movie?"

Now, why do I remember that? It's bizarre how, when your mind and heart are trashed and then, suddenly, you remember the details of a certain event that pushes its way into your mind.

We went outside and it was cold and snowing/raining. The van that Ma was going to ride in was all metal on the inside and very cold. The funeral guy pushed the stretcher in and got everything locked in place. Tom and I each took one of the back doors and again said, "G'bye, Ma," as we closed the doors.

The van drove slowly away, and we watched it, through the wet snowflakes, until it was out of sight.

We went up to her room and I felt out of place; it just didn't seem right to be there without Ma. It's like we were now strangers in a place that had previously been very familiar to us. We gathered a few items and carried them out as we left. In the TV area, it seemed weird that Ma wasn't there in a recliner or curled up on the floor. As we passed through the common area, the trivia game was still in progress. The caregiver looked at me and I waved. She smiled. Then she continued, "This is a fill in the blank question….Who knows the missing name? Larry, blank and Curly."

It was business as usual in the Memory Care unit.

The Three Stooges question stumped the residents for a bit, and it was very quiet. Out of the silence, coming from one of the resident's rooms, I could just barely hear a faint, "My, my, my, my, my…." as the door closed behind us.

EPILOGUE

When my mom and I updated her estate planning documents a few years prior to her dementia diagnosis, she decided that she wanted to be cremated and to have her ashes split between my brothers and I, with a small amount set aside to be scattered in the foothills at the edge of Colorado Springs. She said we didn't need to post an announcement in the obituary section of the local newspaper, and it wasn't necessary to have a formal service of any kind.

We organized a small informal get-together at my house and prior to the gathering Tom, Mai, Sandy and I went to the foothills on a cold Saturday, January 10, 2015. Tom and I had already selected a spot next to a large pinon pine, surrounded by huge, round boulders situated in the red dirt. Tom had a few incense sticks that he lit and stuck in the ground, followed by all of us saying our silent goodbyes as we scattered the ashes around the area. It was a short, somber gathering and when the incense sticks smoldered down to their last wisps, we drove back to my house where our guests were beginning to assemble.

In attendance were my cousin Tim and his wife Anne, a few of Ma's neighbors and a few close friends of ours, along with our daughters. The guests brought small side dishes and snacks, the candles were lit, and soft music played in the background as those of us who were able shared a memory or two of Ma. I was uncharacteristically quiet and only mentioned how, because of Tom, Ma had been able to enjoy a quality of life for her last six months that would never have happened if not for him. We all gave him a nice round of applause, which he surely deserved, and then he had the floor as he shared his thoughts with the group. His topic was about how brave Mom had been when undertaking the many adventures she'd embarked upon during her life. It was very heartfelt and touching and it clearly moved all of us in the room. We then went around the group, not in any particular order, and whoever felt like saying something on Ma's behalf, did so. It was a very sweet and tender occasion, and I'm sure that Ma would have been pleased with how everything worked out.

Over the next several weeks, Tom and Mai went through Ma's house and organized all items that had been promised to various family members along with the even larger inventory that went to Ma's neighbors, our friends, and local donation centers. She wasn't a hoarder by any means, but there was still a whole houseful of stuff to be gone through and sorted. At the end of January, the major share of the work had been completed and we loaded up a large rental truck with the keepsakes bound for Chicagoland. Tom and Mai then headed across the great plains and spent the first few weeks of February at the house of our brother Jim, and his wife Eileen. While there, Tom and Jim organized another informal get-together which was attended by several family members and friends from the Chicago area and from a few of the surrounding states as well. Aunt Mary and Uncle Jim were there of course, as was my Aunt Bernie, along with many of Ma's nieces and nephews, old friends, former neighbors, and coworkers.

At the end of February, Tom and Mai went home to Thailand and we all returned to our lives. It had been a very rough year and a half, and it took all of us, each in our own way, quite some time to work through all that had happened during that period. Another piece of me went away when my mom died, just as it had with my dad and the many other loved ones who had left before her. And life goes on…….

ABOUT THE AUTHOR

John Radzienda lives in Colorado with his wife and two daughters.

He can be reached by email at:

johnradzienda@gmail.com

Made in the
USA
Lexington, KY